OMEGA 3 FATTY ACIDS IN CLINICAL NUTRITION

OMEGA 3 FATTY ACIDS IN CLINICAL NUTRITION

AXEL R. HELLER
S. N. STEHR
AND
T. KOCH
EDITORS

Nova Science Publishers, Inc.
New York

For permission to use material from this book please contact us:
Telephone 631-231-7269; Fax 631-231-8175
Web Site: http://www.novapublishers.com

Library of Congress Cataloging-in-Publication Data

Heller, Axel R.
Omega 3 fatty acids in clinical nutrition / Axel R. Heller and T. Koch.
p. ; cm.
Includes bibliographical references and index.
ISBN 1-59454-601-0
. Omega-3 fatty acids--Physiological effect. 2. Essential fatty acids in human nutrition. I. Koch, Thea. II. Title.
[DNLM: 1. Fatty Acids, Omega-3--physiology. 2. Inflammation--physiopathology. 3. Inflammation Mediators--physiology. 4. Nutrition. QU 90 H477o 2005]
QP752.O44H45 2005
612.3'97--dc22 2005020776

Published by Nova Science Publishers, Inc. ✦ New York

Contents

List of Tables

List of Figures

Acknowledgements

The authors would like to thank Mrs. Dana Niegsch for excellent editorial work and technical assistance, and are indebted to Mrs. Barbara Stehr for her skilled proofreading.

Abbreviations

AA	Arachidonic acid
A_{23185}	Calciumionophore
ARDS	Acute respiratory distress syndrome
COX	Cyclooxygenase
DHA	Docosahexaenoic acid
EFA	Essential fatty acid
EN	Enteral nutrition
EPA	Eicosapentaenoic acid
FO	Fish oil
HEPE	Hydroxyeicosapentaenoic acid
HETE	Hydroxyeicosatetraenoic acid
HPEPE	Hydroperoxy-eicosapentaenoic acid
HPETE	Hydroperoxy-eicosatetraenoic acid
C_{fc}	Capillary filtration coefficient
HDL	High density lipoprotein
HIV	Human immunodeficiency virus
IL	Interleukin
iNOS	Inducible nitric oxide synthase
LDL	Low density lipoprotein
LT	Leukotriene
MARS	Mixed antagonistic response syndrome
MOF	Multiple organ failure
NFκB	Nuclear factor kappa B
NO	Nitric oxide
omega-3 FA	Omega-3-polyunsaturated fatty acids
omega-6 FA	Omega-6-polyunsaturated fatty acids
PAF	Platelet activating factor
PDGF	Platelet derived growth factor
PG	Prostaglandin
PGI_2	Prostacyclin
PLA_2	Phospholipase A_2

RTG	Resonance Thrombography
SAPS II	Simplified acute physiology score II
SIRS	Systemic inflammatory response syndrome
TF	Tissue Factor (cofactor of coagulation factor VII)
TNF	Tumor necrosis factor
TPN	Total parenteral nutrition
TXA_2	Thromboxane A_2
VLDL	Very low density lipoprotein

In: Omega 3 Fatty Acids in Clinical Nutrition
Editors: A. Heller, S. Stehr and T. Koch, pp. 1-4
ISBN 1-59454-601-0

Chapter I

Introduction

Axel R. Heller

During the past decades, intensive collaborative research in the fields of chronic and acute inflammatory disorders has resulted in a better understanding of the pathophysiology and diagnosis of these diseases. Modern therapeutic approaches remain unsatisfactory and shock, sepsis and multiple organ failure (MOF) are still a great challenge in intensive care medicine. Furthermore, treatment of inflammatory diseases like rheumatoid arthritis, ulcerative colitis or psoriasis represents an unresolved problem as well. Many factors contribute to the complex course of inflammatory reactions. Microbiological, immunological and toxic agents are able to initiate the inflammatory response by activating a variety of humoral and cellular mediators. In the early phase of inflammation interleukins and lipid-mediators are excessively released and play a crucial role in the pathogenesis of organ dysfunction.

Cellular lipid membranes represent a dynamic high turnover barrier system, which separates the intracellular from the extracellular space and easily adapts to respective demands. In addition to this barrier function membrane lipids (arachidonic acid) can be oxidized to biologically active lipid mediators (eicosanoids). These function as "local mediators" [9,10] which can quickly reach considerable concentrations and, due to their short half life, act in intercellular microenvironments.

Two omega-3 polyunsaturated fatty acids (omega-3 FA) eicosapentaenoic acid (EPA) and docosahexaenoic acid (DHA) are mainly found in maritime sources, as opposed to omega-6 polyunsaturated fatty acids found in terrestrial sources (the typical western diet). Omega-3 FA such as EPA (C20:5) and DHA (C22:6) can be found in a concentration of 0.1-1.2 % in deep-sea fish [15] and therefore are the main omega-3 FA nutritional reservoir for humans. Historically the intake of saturated fatty acids and unsaturated omega-3 and omega-6 FA has been approximately equal. Contemporary nutritional habits, emphasizing industrially produced vegetable oils and animal fats, have disturbed this balance, resulting in a proportional decrease of omega-3 FA [7].

The first epidemiological studies on omega-3 FA were inspired by the low rate of heart disease among Inuit populations still consuming a traditional diet high in polyunsaturated omega-3 FA. Subsequent studies have established a correlation between the fat content of food and cardiovascular disease, leading to the finding that omega-3 FA can have a beneficial cardiovascular effect [6,7,8]. The intensive research of recent years has also broadened our understanding of just how omega-3 fatty acids work, for instance in promoting the formation of eicosanoids with immunomodulating characteristics.

In states of inflammation, EPA is released from cellular membrane sources to compete with AA for enzymatic metabolism producing less inflammatory and chemotactic derivatives. On the subcellular level omega-3 FA modulate nuclear factor kappa-B derived upregulation of the acute phase response and, thus, prevent overshooting immune response. As a result, improved outcome was observed in a broad range of disease ranging from chronic disorders to cancer and in other critical patient conditions.

The benefits of omega-3 FA, in the form of fish oil, are meanwhile well documented for enteral diets. Diets enriched with omega-3 FA result in a change of the omega-3-/ omega-6-ratio in the membranous fatty acid composition of multiple cells [3,13,17], e.g. erythrocytes [14], neutrophils [4,8], platelets [5,12], endothelial cells, monocytes, brain- [16] and liver cells [2] in favor of pentaenoic acids. On intensive care units with a higher proportion of patients on artificial nutrition, however, one further step is to include omega-3 FA in a concept of immunonutrition. Recent work on clinical nutrition underlined the importance of enteral and parenteral nutrition for patient outcome [1,11,18,19].

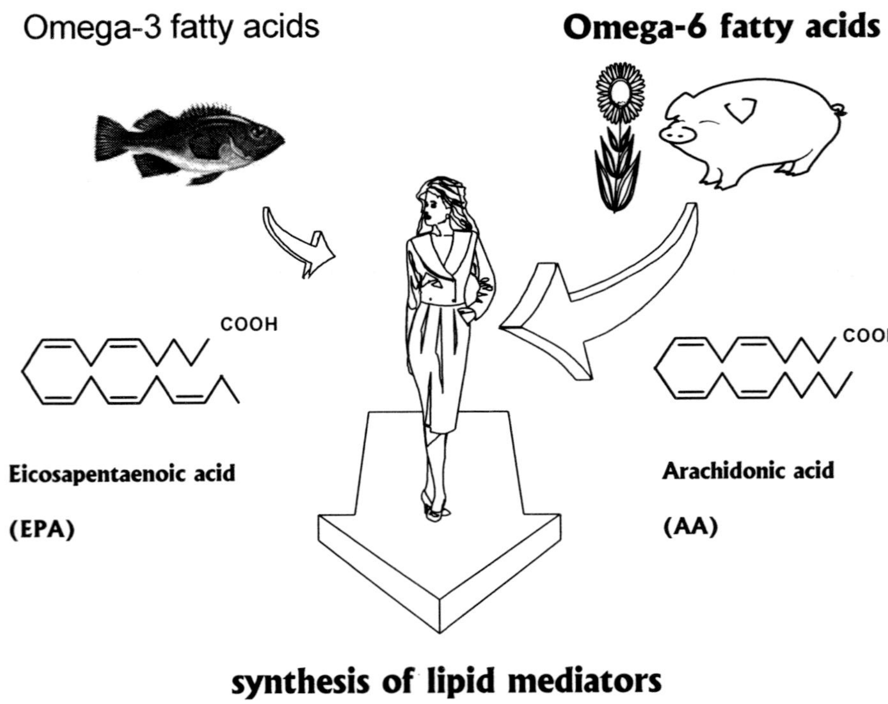

Figure 1. Resources for biogenic fatty acids in industrialized societies

In contrast to numerous studies on the effects of long-term (weeks to months) supplementation with omega-3 FA, more recently the interest has been focused on the question of whether or not omega-3 FA are integrated into the membrane lipid pool even after short-term intravenous application.

Following major abdominal surgery we found that short term intravenous application of omega-3 FA improved liver function without untoward effects on platelet function and coagulation. Moreover, omega-3 FA helped to maintain the balance between pro- and anti-inflammatory cytokines whereby preventing hyper-inflammatory complications. This was confirmed in 661 Patients who received fish oil infusion. Fish oil significantly lowered the occurrence of comorbid infection. Patients whose daily caloric intake included at least 5% fish oil needed fewer antibiotics and had a shorter length of hospital stay. In a multifactor-regression model the two main factors contributing to the length of stay were the amount of omega-6 FA (+1.6d/ 100g) and the delay of nutrition onset (+1.42d/ day of delay).

In view of clinical consequences, these findings show prophylactic and also acute effects in the treatment of inflammatory diseases, which seem easily achieved by a simple rearrangement of nutritional components.

This book aims to give a brief update of the pathophysiological impact of lipid mediators in inflammatory disorders and to summarize the recent development of therapeutic approaches.

References

[1] (2001) Proceedings from Summit on Immune-Enhancing Enteral Therapy. May 25-26, 2000, San Diego, California, USA. *JPEN J.Parenter.Enteral Nutr.* 25:S1-63.

[2] Bourre J. M., Bonneil M., Dumont O., Piciotti M., Calaf R., Portugal H., Nalbone G., Lafont H. (1990) Effect of increasing amounts of dietary fish oil on brain and liver fatty composition. *Biochim.Biophys.Acta* 1043:149-152.

[3] Brown A. J., Pang E., Roberts D. C. (1991) Persistent changes in the fatty acid composition of erythrocyte membranes after moderate intake of n-3 polyunsaturated fatty acids: study design implications. *Am.J.Clin.Nutr.* 54:668-673.

[4] Chilton F. H., Patel M., Fonteh A. N., Hubbard W. C., Triggiani M. (1993) Dietary n-3 fatty acid effects on neutrophil lipid composition and mediator production. Influence of duration and dosage. *J.Clin.Invest* 91:115-122.

[5] Croset M., Bayon Y., Lagarde M. (1992) Incorporation and turnover of eicosapentaenoic and docosahexaenoic acids in human blood platelets in vitro. *Biochem.J.* 281 (Pt 2):309-316.

[6] Dyerberg J.Bang H. O. (1995) Haemostatic function and platelet polyunsaturated fatty acids in Eskimos. 1979. *Nutrition* 11:475-

[7] Dyerberg J., Bang H. O., Hjorne N. (1975) Fatty acid composition of the plasma lipids in Greenland Eskimos. *Am.J.Clin.Nutr.* 28:958-966.

[8] Dyerberg J., Bang H. O., Stoffersen E., Moncada S., Vane J. R. (1978) Eicosapentaenoic acid and prevention of thrombosis and atherosclerosis? *Lancet* 2:117-119.

[9] Heller A., Koch T., Schmeck J., van Ackern K. (1998) Lipid mediators in inflammatory disorders. *Drugs* 55:487-496.

[10] Heller A. R., Theilen H. J., Koch T. (2003) Fish or chips? News Physiol Sci. 18:50-54.

[11] Heyland D. K., Novak F., Drover J. W., Jain M., Su X., Suchner U. (2001) Should immunonutrition become routine in critically ill patients? A systematic review of the evidence. *JAMA* 286:944-953.

[12] Lee T. H., Hoover R. L., Williams J. D., Sperling R. I., Ravalese J., III, Spur B. W., Robinson D. R., Corey E. J., Lewis R. A., Austen K. F. (1985) Effect of dietary enrichment with eicosapentaenoic and docosahexaenoic acids on in vitro neutrophil and monocyte leukotriene generation and neutrophil function. *N.Engl.J.Med.* 312:1217-1224.

[13] Lehr H. A., Hubner C., Finckh B., Nolte D., Beisiegel U., Kohlschutter A., Messmer K. (1991) Dietary fish oil reduces leukocyte/endothelium interaction following systemic administration of oxidatively modified low density lipoprotein. *Circulation* 84:1725-1731.

[14] Seeger W., Wolf H., Stahler G., Neuhof H., Roka L. (1981) [Increase of pulmonary vascular resistance and permeability due to the metabolism of free arachidonic acid (author's transl)]. *Klin.Wochenschr.* 59:459-461.

[15] Simopoulos A. P., Kifer R. R., Martin R. E. (1986) Health effects of polyunsaturated fatty acids in seafood. Academic Press

[16] Tocher D. R., Bell J. G., Sargent J. R. (1991) Incorporation of [3H]arachidonic and [14C]eicosapentaenoic acids into glycerophospholipids and their metabolism via lipoxygenases in isolated brain cells from rainbow trout Oncorhynchus mykiss. *J.Neurochem.* 57:2078-2085.

[17] Urakaze M., Hamazaki T., Makuta M., Ibuki F., Kobayashi S., Yano S., Kumagai A. (1987) Infusion of fish oil emulsion: effects on platelet aggregation and fatty acid composition in phospholipids of plasma, platelets, and red blood cell membranes in rabbits. *Am.J.Clin.Nutr.* 46:936-940.

[18] van den Berghe G., Wouters P., Weekers F., Verwaest C., Bruyninckx F., Schetz M., Vlasselaers D., Ferdinande P., Lauwers P., Bouillon R. (2001) Intensive insulin therapy in the critically ill patients. *N.Engl.J.Med.* 345:1359-1367.

[19] Heller A. R., Rössler S., Litz R. J., Stehr S. N., Heller S. C., Koch T. (2006) Omega-3 fatty acids improve the diagnosis- related clinical outcome. *Crit Care Med.*38:pp

In: Omega 3 Fatty Acids in Clinical Nutrition
Editors: A. Heller, S. Stehr and T. Koch, pp. 5-27
ISBN 1-59454-601-0

Chapter II

Biology of Lipid Mediators and Fatty Acids

Axel R. Heller, Susanne C. Heller and Thea Koch

2.1. Lipid Mediators and the Physiological Inflammation Process

Eicosanoids are "local mediators"[35,36]. They are generated in various tissues and cells e.g. lung, liver, kidney or neutrophils, and tend to ensue their effects locally because of their short half-life due to quick enzymatic inactivation. Therefore the measured systemic levels of lipid mediators must be considered as a "spill over", and do not allow estimations about local concentrations.

Lipid mediators are a fundamental part of the complex processes leading to the main signs of inflammation. The inflammatory reaction is characterized by the stimulation of humoral and cellular mediator systems and the release of a great variety of inflammatory mediators, which result in alterations in microvascular tone and permeability. Lipid mediators are essentially involved in the regulation of these complex actions. Prostaglandins such as PGE_2 and PGI_2 support the formation of an inflammatory edema (tumor), through their vasodilative properties (rubor), and contribute to the development of hyperalgesia at the site of inflammation (dolor). Fatty acid peroxides and leukotrienes additionally increase the local permeability and are potent chemo-attractants for neutrophil granulocytes resulting in a further microcirculatory accumulation of phagocytes. Platelet activating factor (PAF) is another important lipid mediator, which maintains inflammatory activity by stimulation of neutrophils [35,36] and partially influences the vascular tone and permeability. Besides that, PAF is a chemotactic agent, which contributes to leukocyte-mediated injury in inflammatory processes.

The precursors for all lipid mediators, therefore, are fatty acids as a part of cellular lipid membranes. In particular, arachidonic acid, a fourfold polyunsaturated fatty acid consisting of 20 carbon atoms is a fundamental part of membrane lipids.

Arachidonic acid (AA) is the mother substance of the pro-inflammatory eicosanoids. It is released from membrane phospholipids in the course of inflammation by phospholipases and is metabolized to prostaglandins and leukotrienes.

2.2. The Eicanosoid Pathway

Unsaturated fatty acids are divided into mono- and polyunsaturated fatty acids (figure 2). From the first double bound in the polyunsaturated fatty acid on, regarded from the methyl end, the FA are further divided into omega-3, omega-6 and omega-9 FA. Oleic acid (C18:1) is a monounsaturated fatty acid, which can be synthesized by mammalians, whereas omega-3 and omega-6 FA are essential for humans [10,14]. Omega-6 FA, such as linoleic acid (C18:2) and AA (C20:4) are found in plant oils and fatty tissues of mammalians, which represent the major part of FAs in the diet of industrialized societies. In individuals without relevant dietary intake of omega-3 FA, AA is predominantly released from the phospholipid pool of cellular membranes, which is metabolized by two major pathways to pro-inflammatory mediators [87].

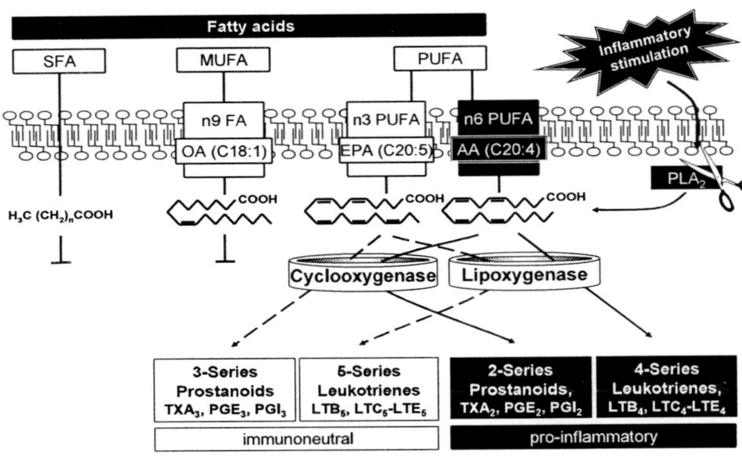

Figure 2. Eicosanoid pathways. Depending on the fatty acid content of cellular membranes lipid mediators are generated from omega-3- or omega-6-polyunsatureated fatty acids (PUFA) via the cyclo- or lipoxygenase pathway. The arachidonic acid- (AA) metabolites leukotrienes (LT) and thrmboxane (TX) A_2 with pro-inflammatory and eicosapentaenoic acid- (EPA) derivatives with reduced inflammatory properties. The mono unsaturated fatty acid (MUFA) oleic acid (OA) and saturated fatty acids (SFA) without relevant inflammatory mediator generation (Reprinted with permission of the American Physiologic Society, from Heller AR, et al., News Physiol Sci 2003)

In case of inflammation the activation of membrane-linked phospholipase A_2 (PLA_2) induces the mobilization of fatty acids, particularly AA from membrane lipids.The vaso- and broncho-constrictive metabolites thromboxane (TX) A_2 and prostaglandin (PG) $F_{2\alpha}$ are produced via the cyclooxygenase-pathway. The TXA_2 induced vaso- and bronchospasm predominates the relaxing effects of simultaneously generated prostacyclin (PGI_2) and PGE_2 on smooth muscle cells of vessels and bronchioli. The pattern of eicosanoids depends on the enzyme content of the particular cells [35,36,64]. While TXA_2 is produced mainly in platelets and macrophages, PGI_2 is derived from endothelial cells. PGE_2 is predominantly synthesized in the renal medulla. Mastcells are the main source for PGD_2.

In addition to the described cyclooxygenase pathway, AA is also metabolized via the lipoxygenase-pathway forming the leukotrienes (LTB_4, LTC_4, LTD_4, LTE_4) and other eicosanoids, which increase capillary permeability and attract neutrophils via chemotactic properties [76]. LTB_4 is produced in neutrophils and macrophages, while eosinophils and mast cells form LTC_4, LTD_4 and LTE_4 [92,96].

2.3. Omega-3 Fatty Acids

2.3.1. Origin of Omega-3 Fatty Acids

The development of the human species began almost 4 million years ago. Man developed within a defined nutritional environment and the nutritional fatty acid composition affected man's adaptation to his biologic niche, regarding body and brain size, metabolic rate, and host defense including the inflammatory process itself (figure 3).

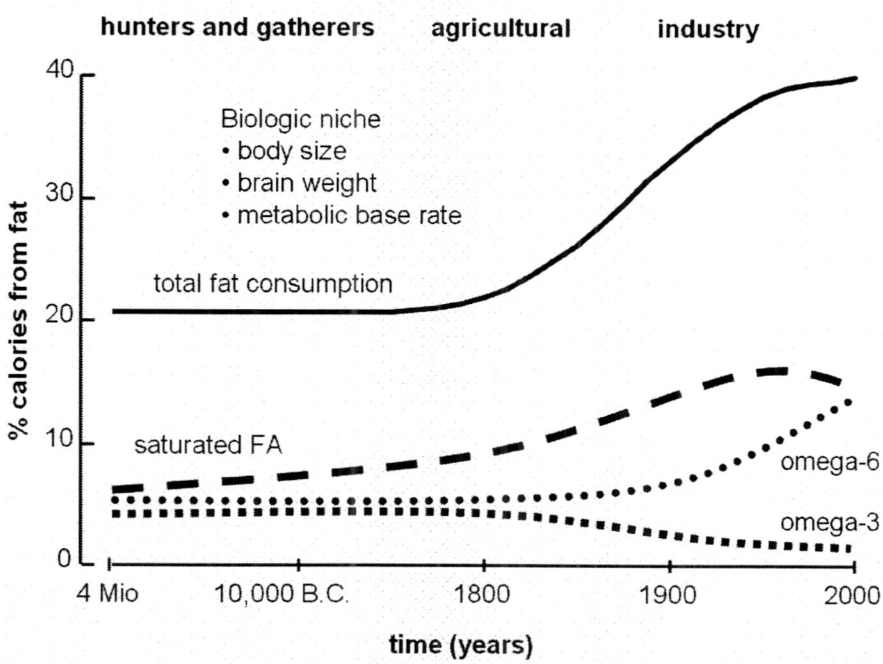

Figure 3. Human nutritional development. While mankind developed into its unique biologic niche in a nutritional environment of equally distributed omega-6 to omega-3 ratios (0.1-2.8) industrial nutrition habits increased the omega-6/omega-3 ratio to 3.3- 16.7.

Contemporary nutritional habits, emphasizing the consumption of industrially produced vegetable oils and animal fats, have disturbed this balance, resulting in a proportional decrease of omega-3 FA. Therefore, inflammatory cascades use substrates that are not actually part of the developmental design of the defense system.Today omega-6 FA, such as linolenic acid (C18:2 omega-6) and AA (C20:4 omega-6), which can be found in vegetable oils and in the fat depot of mammals, make up the largest part of the fatty acid intake of industrialized societies. Studies of the cell membrane structure of these populations, thus, show a predominance of omega-6 FA. In contrast, communities with a major intake of deep-sea fish incorporate larger quantities of polyunsaturated omega-3 FA into cellular membranes, leading to a proportional reduction of omega-6 FA.

Long-chain omega-3 FA such as eicosapentaenoic acid (EPA) and docosahexaenoic acid (DHA) are produced in algae and plankton. Plankton is the main source of nutrition for deep-sea fish (e.g. herring, salmon, mackerel, tuna, and sardines) and their fish oils provide the main source of omega-3 FA for humans. In deep-sea fish EPA (C20:5 omega-3) and DHA (C22:6 omega-3) can be found in concentrations of 0.1–1.2% [81]. The human organism is only capable of synthesizing small amounts of EPA from α-linolenic acid. [10,14].

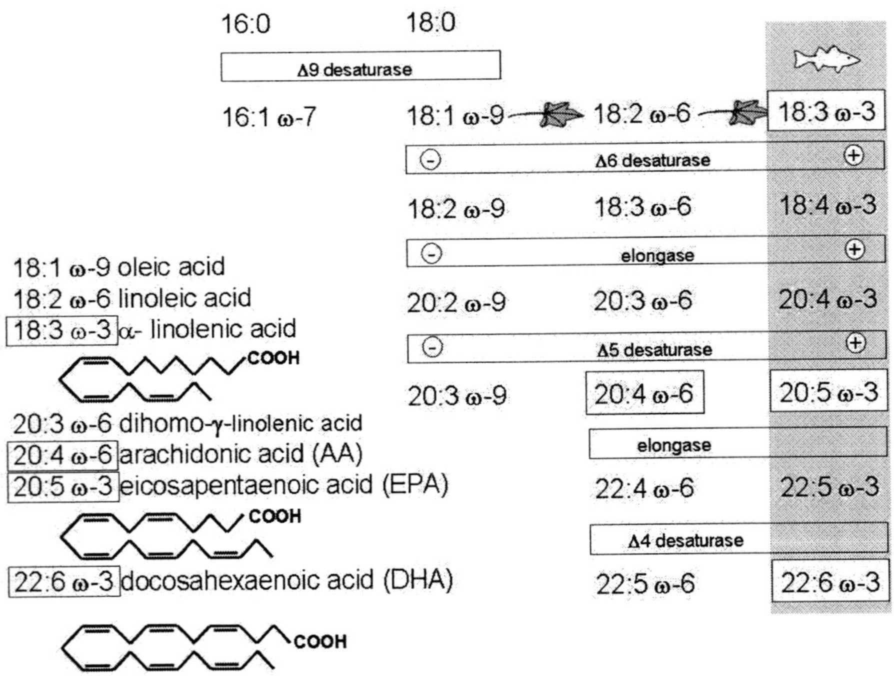

Figure 4. Overview over the synthesis cascade of polyunsaturated fatty acids within plants and fish. Arachidonic acid (AA) eicosapentaenoic acid (EPA); docosahexaenoic acid (DHA). Substrate affinity of enzymes (-) = low; (+) = high (Figures translated, modified, and reprinted with permission of Georg Thieme Publishers, Stuttgart, Germany, from Heller AR, et al., AINS 1998)

How can omega-3 FA become a part of a daily diet? The structures of the main omega-3 FA are shown in figure 4. Alpha-linolenic acid is the mother substance of the long chain omega-3-FA EPA and DHA. Vegetable oil, especially linseed oil is the major source of α-linolenic acid.

Biochemical pathways for omega-3 desaturation exist only in chloroplasts; meaning only algae and plankton are capable of forming those essential fatty acids (EFA) in relevant amounts. Human cells are unable to introduce double bonds in positions prior to carbon 9 counting from the omega terminus. Therefore, all three omega-3 FA are an essential part of the human diet. Marine plants such as algae and plankton are the primary source of EFA in the marine food chain. Fish that live off plankton are able to elongate and desaturate the parent EFA, forming long-chain poly unsaturated FA. Direct consumption of deep-sea fish is a simple method of including omega-3 FA in a daily diet. The amount of omega-3 FA per 100g of fish varies from one species to another. Mackerels have the highest content of omega-3 FA with 2.2 g / 100 g body weight. In addition herring, salmon and tuna have high concentrations of omega-3 FA (see Table 1). One must of course bear in mind the high cholesterol concentration found in these species.

Table 1. Omega-3 FA content of different fish

Fish	Fatty acids [g/100g]				
	20:5	22:6	Total omega-3-content	Cholesterol [mg/100g]	Chol./ ω-3-FA
Mackerel, king	1.0	1.2	2.2	53	0.024
Herring, Pacific	1.0	0.7	1.7	77	0.045
Anchovy	0.5	0.9	1.4	51	0.036
Salmon, chinook	0.8	0.6	1.4	58	0.041
Tuna, albacore	0.3	1.0	1.3	54	0.042
Salmon, pink	0.4	0.6	1.0	51	0.051
Halibut, Greenland	0.5	0.4	0.9	46	0.051

The daily requirement of omega-6 linoleic acid is 4-5g, while the amount of polyunsaturated omega-3 FA is rougly half of that (table 2). However, the requirement may substantially increase under deficiency and during critical illness. As part of a normal diet and under physiological conditions the minimal requirement of omega-3 FA can be achieved by eating two meals of fish (each including 100-200g of fish) which contain a high percentage of omega-3 FA per week.

Table 2. Daily requirements of fatty acids in a 2,000 kcal diet, according to [81]

Fatty acid	g/d	% energy
linoleic acid (omga-6)	4.44	2.0
α-linolenic acid (omega-3)	2.22	1.0
EPA + DHA (omega-3)	0.65	0.3

After the publication of the first positive results of large controlled studies several commercial pharmaceutical companies marketed capsules containing fish oil with standardized amounts of omega-3 FA. A standard recommended dose of two capsules daily is equal to 660 mg of omega-3 FA. Since the value of fish oil in health and during disease conditions was widely recognized, the fishing industry is confronted with an increased demand for fish by the consumers.

The large commercial fishing industry, however, substantially endangers various species of the deep-sea fish population. Especially salmon and tuna populations have been depleted and some tuna species are listed as endangered. In fact, most of the salmon offered today is bred and contains not only beneficial omega-3 FA, but also toxic substances and traces of antibiotics. Tuna fishing has developed into a highly specialized industry, systematically reducing the fish's natural habitat. The number of other species (i.e. sharks and turtles) endangered by this fishing method is immense and remains a major concern of environmentalist organizations. Herring and mackerels with large amounts of omega-3 FA travel in large shoals which makes for an easy catch containing a low amount of additional fish species. Moreover, cost-use calculations suggest using the latter species due to their relative high amount of omega-3 FA. Considering that consumption of one to two servings of mackerel or herring per week covers the human demand for omega-3 FA at present these species may serve as a reasonable ecological source of omega-3 FA.

2.3.2. Effects of Omega-3 Fatty Acids on the Eicosanoid Pathway

In case of increased membrane lipid content of omega-3 FA, EPA competes with AA for metabolization via the cyclo- and lipoxygenase pathway [23,84,88]. The EPA- derived metabolites have lower a biological activity [53,63], compared to the analogous AA-derivatives (figure 5). While AA is metabolized by cyclooxygenase to diene prostanoids (prostaglandins and thromboxane), by lipoxygenase to 4 series-leukotrienes (tetraenoic leukotrienes) and hydroxyeicosatetraenoic acids (HETE), EPA is converted to triene-prostanoids by cyclooxygenase. In comparison with the AA-derived TXA_2, the EPA-derived cyclooxygenase-product of the 3-series TXA_3 has considerably reduced pro-aggregatory and vasoconstrictive properties, while PGI_3 possesses similar anti-aggregatory and vasodilative effects as PGI_2. Moreover, EPA represents a preferred substrate of 5-lipoxygenase [52,68]. After the enzymatic conversion of EPA, the 5-series leukotrienes (LTB_5, C_5, D_5, E_5) are generated, which, compared to AA-derivatives, have partially antagonistic biologic effects [54,93]. The vasoconstrictive and chemotactic potency of LTB_5 is two orders of magnitude lower than the activity of LTB_4 [15,30]. In addition, the generation of pro-inflammatory PAF is reduced by EPA via interference with the PAF precursor-pool [83,86].

Depending on the enzyme pattern of the respective cell (e.g. thrombocytes, endothelial cells, leukocytes, etc.) these fatty acids are turned into endoperoxides by enzyme cyclooxygenase, from which prostaglandins, prostacyclins and thromboxanes are formed. Lipoxygenase primarily creates hydroperoxides and subsequently leukotrienes [94]. The derivatives formed from EPA are different from the analogous AA derivatives in structure and biological activity [35].

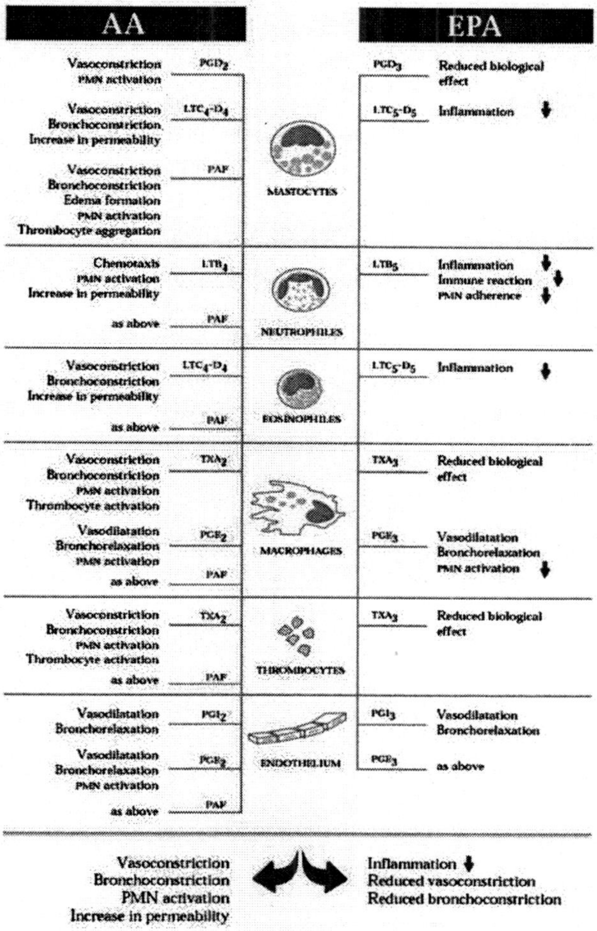

Figure 5. Overview over the profiles of action of different Lipid mediators derived from omega-6-arachidonic (AA) and omega-3 eicosapentaenoic acid (EPA) and their respective sites of synthesis. (Translated and reprinted with permission of Georg Thieme Publishers, Stuttgart, Germany, from Heller AR, et al., Zentralbl. Chir 2000)

2.3.3. Signal Transduction Effects of Omega-3 Fatty Acids

Apart from supplying energy, polyunsaturated omega-3 FA exert immune modulating and organ protective effects [35,36]. Depending on the nutritional intake, omega-3 FA are incorporated in the phospholipid pool of cellular membranes and replace the omega-6 FA, thereby increasing membrane fluidity and influencing lipid mediator and cytokine production [6,56],

While the impact of omega-3 FA on lipid mediator generation has been fully clarified, the understanding of subcellular effects remains, at this time, limited. Omega-3 FA affect biophysical characteristics of cellular membranes by altering the membrane phospholipid composition and the content of cholesterol, thereby improving membrane fluidity. The associated increase in the deformability of blood cells may account for improvements of blood rheology after fish oil intake. Furthermore, omega-3 FA modify the function of membrane-linked enzyme systems, signal transducing and receptor functions. Recent work by Lee and coworkers demonstrated that the activation of general pro-inflammatory pathways, such as NFκB and cyclooxygenase-2 expression by saturated fatty acids and the inhibition of this induction by polyunsaturated fatty is mediated through a common signaling pathway derived from the toll-like receptor (TLR)-4 [51]. As a part of innate immunity TLR-4 conveys signals from the endotoxin receptor (CD14) on the surface of macrophages to the inner cell and may, likewise, be activated by saturated fatty acids. In addition, TLR-2 is activated by cell surface components of gram-positive bacteria, which may be blunted by omega-3 FA.

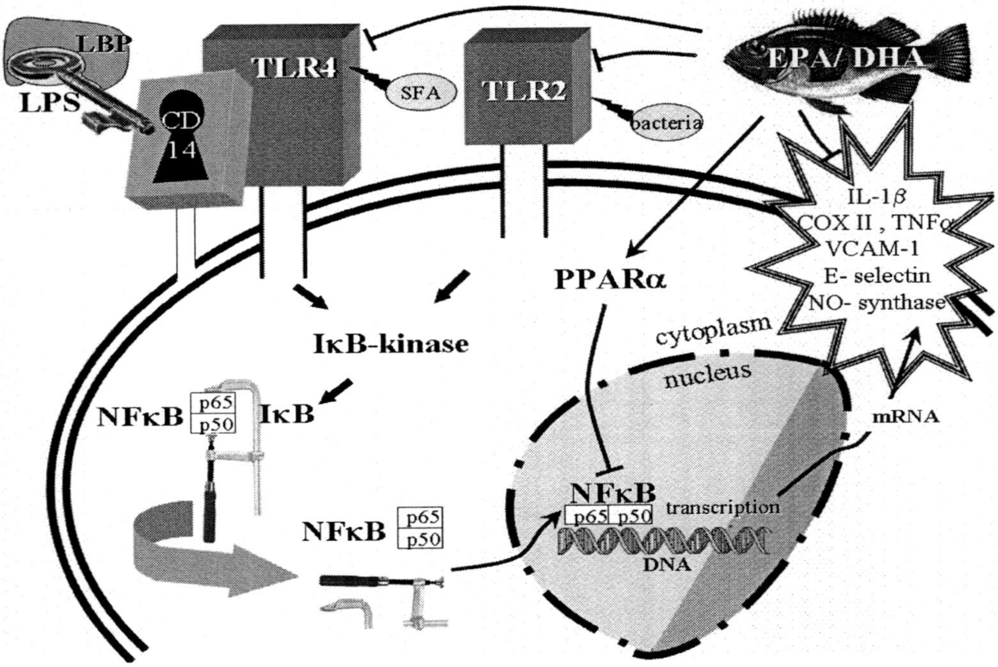

Figure 6. Effects of omega 3 fatty acids on the toll like receptor (TLR)- nuclear factor kappa B (NFκB)- axis. While TLR-4 confers the presence of a gram-negative infection to the inner cell, TLR-2 reports the presence of gram-positive bacteria. Saturated fatty acids (SFA) may, likewise, activate the TLR-4 cascade. Via IκB-kinase the blockade- function of inhibitory factor kappa B (IκB) is postponed and NFκB may translocate into the nucleus to setup transcription activity of inflammatory DNA-gene loci. Consequently inflammatory receptors, enzymes, and cytokines are expressed; Omega-3 eicosapentaenoic acid (EPA) and docosahexaenoic acid (DHA) may competitively interfere into the activating sequence on various levels of the cascade; lipoid binding protein (LBP), lipopolysaccharide (LPS); peroxisome proliferator-activated receptor (PPAR)

As figure 6 shows omega-3 FA modify cellular receptor functions [50] and downstream signal transduction features [77] to the level of NFκB and beyond [7,66]. As a result of the down regulation of nuclear transcription factors formation of cytokines such as TNFα and IL-1 [60] in monocytes are reduced after fish oil. Thus, omega-3-FA seem to interfere with early inflammatory signal transduction processes and may prevent hyper-inflammatory states. A large body of experimental data confirms that omega-3 FA attenuate an overwhelming inflammatory reaction [44], ameliorate host defense [42,91], improve splanchnic blood flow and gut barrier function [69] in septic states, and prevent tumor growth [21]. These different biologic properties of omega-3 FA offer promising prophylactic and therapeutic potentials in different clinical settings which seem to be attainable by supplementing parenteral nutrition with omega-3 FA even after short term administration [56].

2.3.4. Systemic Effects of Omega-3 Fatty Acids

In addition to their effects on lipid mediator formation, omega-3 FA are capable of altering cellular functions which are determined by physical characteristics of biomembranes such as the composition of phospholipids and the content of cholesterol [27]. Omega-3 FA modify the function of membrane-linked enzyme systems, signal transduction [1,17,82] and receptor function [67,74]. The release of IL-1 and TNFα influenced by omega-3 FA could alter the virus replication rate of HIV, as it has been postulated in humans [70,90]. Moreover it has been reported that the expression of certain oncogenes is modulated by omega-3 FA [22]. Especially, anti-arteriosclerotic effects of omega-3 FA have been closely investigated. Although numerous trials analyzing the profile of plasma lipids show in part different results, long term intake of 2-6g/d fish oil seems to be capable of lowering the plasma-triglyceride levels, while HDL slightly increases, and LDL as well as cholesterol remain constant or even decrease slightly [31,49,57]. During the acute phase response omega-3 FA may prevent a fall of HDL levels, which were shown to negatively correlate with outcome. Moreover VLDL-levels may increase due to improvements of the liver function (see chapter 3.4).

The correlation between high plasma lipid concentrations and the development of arteriosclerosis is well known. In this context it was shown, that a fish oil diet reduced intima hyperplasia [48] and coronary sclerosis [89]. Sacks and coworkers published controversial data, which showed no changes in the angiographic determined coronary diameters after a 2-year intake of 6 g daily [72]. In other patient studies diets containing omega-3 FA resulted in reduced rates of restenosis after percutanous transluminal coronary angioplasty (PTCA), [12,28]. Within the scope of diabetic vascular occlusive disease [4,74] and neuropathies [8] omega-3 FA had a protective effect on the vessel wall and improved rheology [34], along with an improved metabolic situation. These findings could be attributed to the reduced formation of platelet-derived growth factor (PDGF) from the vascular endothelium after a diet containing omega-3 FA [24], or the increased release of "endothelium derived relaxing factor" nitric oxide (NO) [80]. NO in combination with vasodilative prostaglandins [11,79] supports the relaxation of the artery's smooth muscle and of resistance vessels.

In a small number of studies omega-3 FA were used as a therapy for arterial hypertension [62], which revealed controversial results. While some investigators report a dose-dependent decrease of blood pressure, others conclude that omega-3 FA do not influence blood pressure. The EPA-doses (up to 15 g/d) used in the therapy of mild hypertension resulted in a decrease of blood pressure by 3-6.5 mmHg [61,79].

2.4. Interventions in Lipid Mediation

Various strategies have been evaluated attempting to control the excessive production of lipid mediators on different levels of biochemical pathways such as inhibition of phospholipase A_2, the trigger-enzyme for AA-release, the blockade of cyclooxygenase- and lipoxygenase pathway as well as the development of receptor antagonists against platelet-activating factor and leukotrienes. Some of these agents exerted protective effects in different inflammatory disorders like septic organ failure, rheumatoid arthritis or asthma, whereas others failed to do so.

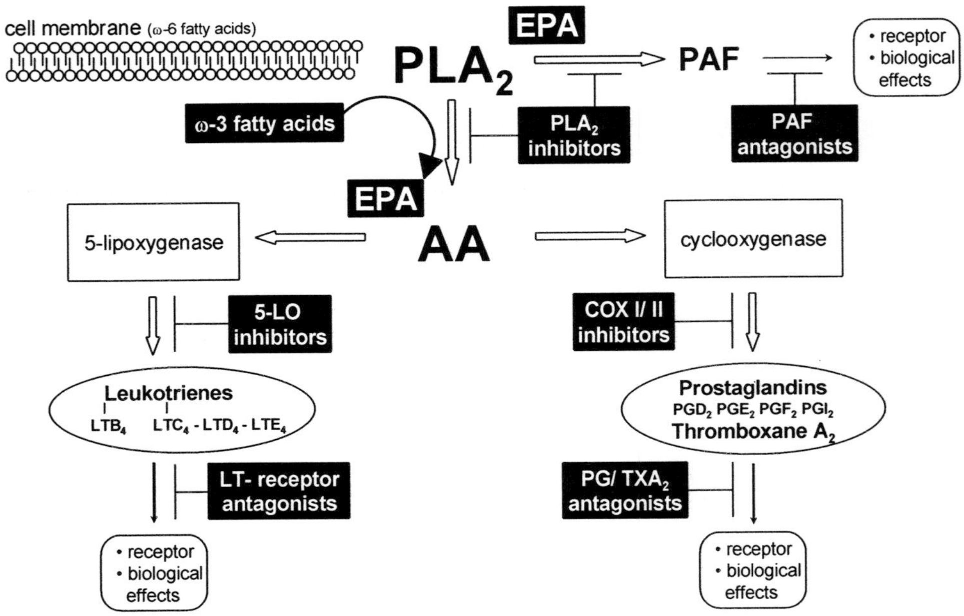

Figure 7. Overview of possibilities to inhibit the lipid mediator pathway (white boxes), interventions black boxes [35]. (Reprinted with permission of Adis International Ltd. Wolters Kluwer Health, Auckland, New-Zealand, from Heller AR, et al., Drugs 1998; 55(4) 487-96)

2.4.1. Prostaglandins

A variety of substances that inhibit the cyclooxygenase pathway have been investigated including non-steroidal anti-inflammatory drugs (NSAIDs). These are commonly used in the treatment of inflammation, pain and fever. Over twenty-five NSAIDs are currently available. These compounds are believed to act via an inhibition of the enzyme cyclooxygenase (COX), which catalyzes the conversion of AA to the prostaglandins and thromboxane (figure 7). Although available NSAIDs are efficacious anti-inflammatory agents, serious side effects limit their use. Two forms of COX were identified, a constitutively expressed COX-1 and a cytokine inducible COX-2. It has been suggested that NSAID-toxicity is due to an inhibition of COX-1, whereas therapeutic properties derive from COX-2-inhibition at the site of the inflammation [47,75]. Therefore selective COX-2 inhibitors such as SC-58125 may exert anti-inflammatory effects without gastrointestinal toxicity [2]. In recent clinical trials the efficacy of COX-2 inhibitors in the therapy of arthritis was evaluated pointing towards sufficient symptom relief with an improved gastrointestinal tolerability [26]. Moreover there is growing evidence that COX-2 inhibition could suppress growth of colorectal cancer [78].

Table 3. Effects of COX-1 and 2.

COX-1 preference	**COX-2 preference/specificity**	**Effects:**
Piroxicam Sulindac Acetylsalicylic acid Indomethacin Ibuprofen	Diclofenac Meloxicam NS398 L-745,337 SC-58125 Clecoxib Parecoxib Rofecoxib Valdecoxib	• Improvement of: Pain, edema, fever, tachycardia, O2 consumption, lactacidosis • Reduction of: platelet aggregation mucosal PG production (COX-1 inhibition) colorectal cancer growth (COX-2 inhibition)

(Reprinted with permission of Adis International Ltd. Wolters Kluwer Health, Auckland, New-Zealand, from [35])

Anti- inflammatory concepts based upon COX-2 selective coxibs recently had to face a considerable drawback, when they were reported to cause severe cardiovascular side effects and, consequently, two out of six formerly approved COX-2 inhibitors were withdrawn from the market [98].

Studies investigating the effect of COX inhibitors in septic conditions demonstrated that ibuprofen was able to attenuate most of the adverse consequences of endotoxin administration and to prolong survival in an animal model [58]. Bernhard et al. lately reported reduced levels of PGI_2 and thromboxane in septic patients after administration of ibuprofen. Fever, tachycardia, oxygen consumption and lactacidosis were improved, whereas the development of shock and ARDS or the mortality rate were unaltered [5]. While ibuprofen not only inhibits such inflammatory COX-products as thromboxane but also the vasodilator PGI_2, another interesting approach is the inhalative application of PGI_2 in the therapy of acute respiratory distress to improve the ventilation-perfusion ratio (V/Q) in the lung [97]. Aerosolized PGI_2 selectively induces pulmonary vasodilation and redistribution of blood flow from shunted areas to well ventilated regions thereby increasing oxygenation in severe ARDS [97]. It appears that PGI_2 is a valuable tool in the therapy of V/Q-mismatch. The beneficial as well as the adverse effects of COX- inhibition suggest a combination of systemic COX 2- inhibition and the additional inhalative PGI_2 supplementation in acute lung failure.

A further approach to selectively reduce COX-induced vasoconstriction and platelet aggregation without a blockade of PGI_2 is to antagonize TXA_2 synthesis. In a model of coronary thrombosis Guth and coworkers demonstrated anti-thrombotic properties of DTTX30, a combined TXA_2 receptor antagonist and synthase inhibitor [32]. Thus, the exclusive inhibition of TXA_2 generation might be a helpful tool in preventing vasoconstriction and platelet aggregation.

2.4.2. Leukotrienes

Leukotrienes (LT) are potent pro-inflammatory agents involved in the pathophysiology of various inflammatory diseases such as asthma, psoriasis, rheumatoid arthritis, and ulcerative colitis [33]. Therefore, many anti-leukotriene compounds have been developed which selectively block either receptor sites or enzymes related to their biosynthesis. A synopsis of these drugs and their effects is given in table 4. Both categories of agents have been shown to decrease bronchial obstruction in asthma [40,85], suggesting that leukotrienes and the 5-lipoxygenase products of arachidonic acid are involved in sustaining the acute airway response that occurs after bronchial provocation in patients with mild to moderate asthma. Leukotriene antagonists and 5-lipoxygenase inhibitors seem to be promising therapeutic tools but they are unlikely to dominate the further therapy of asthma. One of the main considerations in favor of their use is that they can be given orally [41]. Nickerson-Nutter demonstrated the efficacy of the combination of leukotriene synthesis inhibitors and cyclooxygenase inhibitors in models of rheumatoid arthritis [65]. With regard to the chemotactic properties of LTB_4 specific receptor antagonists have been designed to control LTB_4 effects.

Table 4. Effects of leukotriene receptor antagonists and 5-lipoxygenase inhibitors:

Leukotriene receptor antagonists	5-lipoxygenase-inhibitors	Improvement of
Cinalukast ICI204219 L648,051 L649,923 LY293111 MK571 ONO1078 (Pranlukast) Pobilukast edamine RG12525 SC41930 Singulair SKF104353 Tomelukast Verlukast Zafirlukast	A64077 (Zileuton) Bayx1005 BW755C ICI211,965 ICID2138 (ZD2138) MK0591 MK885 Piripost R68151 RS43179	• asthmatic reaction to inhaled LTs and PAF • bronchoconstriction • peak flow rate • forced expiratory volume • symptoms of asthma • rhinitis/ rhinorhea • global disease scores in psoriasis • symptoms of inflammatory bowel disease • reduced requirement of β_2 agonists

(Reprinted with permission of Adis International Ltd. Wolters Kluwer Health, Auckland, New-Zealand, from [35])

It has been demonstrated that LY293111 reduces the upregulation of MAC-1 which plays an important role in neutrophil adhesion [55]. Moreover this LTB_4-receptor antagonist decreased the number of neutrophils in bronchoalveolar lavage fluid of patients with allergen sensitive asthma [20]. LTB_4 antagonism could be a therapeutic approach in LTB_4-dependent disorders, such as ulcerative colitis or psoriasis. Until now, no data is available concerning the use of these agents in septic patients. Whether the inhibition of LT might be useful as a strategy for controlling pro-inflammatory lipid mediators has to be assessed in future clinical studies.

2.4.3. Phospholipase A_2 (PLA_2)

Activation of the PLA_2 is a key step in the production of precursors for the biosynthesis of inflammatory lipid mediators. Inhibition of this enzyme could result in the suppression of three important classes of inflammatory lipids, (prostaglandins, leukotrienes and platelet activating factor) and offers an attractive therapeutic approach to design novel agents for the treatment of inflammation and tissue injury. The phospholipase A_2 family is a series of enzymes involved in the phospholipid catabolism. More than 150 PLA_2 amino acid sequences are currently available in protein sequence databases. PLA_2 exists in both extracellular and intracellular forms. Secretory PLA_2 ($sPLA_2$) are Ca^{2+} dependent enzymes (MW: 14 kDa, regulated by millimol [Ca^{2+}] which are classified in two groups based on their primary structures [3]. Secretory non-pancreatic PLA_2 has been implicated in the pathogenesis of articular inflammation in rheumatoid arthritis, whereas pancreatic PLA_2 contributes to the tissue damage associated with acute pancreatitis. The cytosolic PLA_2 ($cPLA_2$) is a 85,2 kDa enzyme with a substrate specificity for arachidonic acid. It is found in most cells and tissues and is regulated by Ca^{2+} in micromolar range [46]. $cPLA_2$ plays an important role both in rapid and prolonged cellular responses occuring during inflammatory processes. Accordingly, in previous years it has been proposed to use PLA_2 inhibitors in the control of inflammatory diseases. A tremendous number of inhibitors have been claimed as inhibitors of PLA_2 activity. PLA_2 inhibitors are currently investigated using classical inflammatory models [29]. Table 5 shows selected inhibitory agents with marked in vivo activity. For adequate treatment it has been found necessary to apply a cell-impermeable PLA_2 inhibitor, which affects cell membrane activity but does not enter the cell. Yedgar et al. [95] demonstrated improvement in bleomycin-induced lung injury in hamsters after treatment with carboxymethylcellulose linked phosphatidylethanolamine. To date only a few interventional studies with PLA_2 antagonists have been performed. Baboons which were immunized with a neutralizing monoclonal anti PLA_2-II antibody showed significantly attenuated hypotension after treatment with viable E.coli [73]. Moreover, lung vascular leakage in rats due to gut ischemia and reperfusion was blunted [45].

In discussing phospholipase A_2 inhibition it must be kept in mind that not only the formation of subsequent pro-inflammatory lipid mediators is prevented but also the generation of thrombo-regulatory, vasodilative and anti-aggregatory PGI_2 and PGE_2. To what extent PLA_2 inhibitors will reach therapeutical significance in inflammatory diseases has to be elucidated in further clinical studies.

Table 5. Phospholipase A_2 inhibitors and their inhibitory effects

Inhibitors	Reported inhibition of
Natural compounds:	
• Steroids • Lipocortin-1 • Manoalide • BMS-181162 • Scalaradial • Aristolochic acid • YM-26567-1 • YM-26734 • Thilocin A1β • Thilocin B3	• In vitro: PLA_2 I + II • In vivo: Phorbolester- and PLA_2-induced skin inflammation Edema and cellular infiltration
Synthetic compounds:	
• 3-acrylic acid derivatives • Dehydroabietylamine derivatives • WAY-121,520	• In vitro: PLA_2 II • In vivo: Rat paw edema Eicosanoid formation Phorbolester- induced ear edema Bronchospasm

(with permission of Adis International Ltd. Wolters Kluwer Health, Auckland, New- Zealand, from [35])

2.4.4. Platelet Activating Factor (PAF)

The platelet activating factor, a PLA_2 dependent phospholipid is an extraordinarily potent mediator of shock [38] and inflammation. It exerts its biologic effects by activating the PAF receptor and, subsequently, stimulating protein kinase C and increasing intracellular Ca^{2+}. PAF is found in most biologic fluids and is synthesized in most cell types (figures 5). Microvascular permeability is markedly increased by PAF, allowing fluids to leak out of the circulation. Concerning hemodynamic effects, PAF is negative inotropic and lowers arterial blood pressure. It is a potent platelet aggregator and leukocyte activator, and it strongly promotes AA-metabolism. It has been proposed to play a crucial role in the pathogenesis of rheumatoid arthritis, asthma, endotoxin shock and acute renal transplant rejection. In animal models PAF caused bronchoconstriction and increased airway resistance, pulmonary hypertension, and gastrointestinal ulceration. Due to the problem of selective PAF inhibition on the PLA_2 level a variety of PAF receptor antagonists were used in animal models of sepsis with promising results as depicted in table 6 [9,18]. Anti-inflammatory effects of PAF antagonists on experimental models of arthritis have been published [59] indicating the modulation of different pro-inflammatory cytokines. Data obtained in a model of immune-complex arthritis demonstrated controversial regulatory effects of the PAF antagonist WEB

2170 on eicosanoid release. Whereas PGE_2 and TNF levels dropped, LTB_4 release was increased [71]. A clinical trial carried out by Hilliquin and coworkers revealed improvement of rheumatoid arthritis after using another PAF receptor antagonist BN50730 [37].

Table 6. Inhibiors of platelet activating factor and effects.

Inhibitors of Platelet activating factor and reported inhibitory effects
Natural compounds:
• Terpens Ginkolids A, B, C, M, J: Platelet and Leukocyte aggregation, hypotension, edema, vasoconstriction, cardiovascular and renal effects • Lignans Kadsurenone: Platelet aggregation, hypotension, bronchoconstriction, cardial effects, leukocyte degranulation • Gliotoxins FR900452: Platelet aggregation FR49175: Bronchoconstriction
Synthetic compounds:
• Structurally related to PAF e.g. CV3988, SRI27417, ONO6240, RO19-3704: Platelet aggregation, hypotension, endotoxin shock, bronchoconstriction, edema, gastric ulceration, LPS-induced lung injury • Unrelated to PAF structure Thiazolderivatives e.g. RP 48740, RP52629: Platelet aggregation hypotension, bronchospasm, hyperfibrinolysis, gastric ulceration Thiazolobenzodiazepines e.g. WEB2086, BN50730, RO15-1788, TCV307: Shock induced immunosuppression, bronchoconstriction, platelet and leukocyte aggregation, edema, hypotension, anaphylaxis, gastric ulceration, cytokine release, rheumatoid arthritis

(Reprinted with permission of Adis International Ltd. Wolters Kluwer Health, Auckland, New-Zealand, from [35])

Dhainhaut et al. [13] performed a placebo-controlled double blind study including 262 patients with sepsis syndrome. In addition to their standard supportive therapy patients received the PAF-receptor antagonist BN52021 twice daily (120mg) over four days or a placebo, respectively. The overall 28-day mortality in the BN52021 group did not differ significantly from the placebo group but in the subgroup of gram-negative sepsis BN52021 significantly reduced mortality (57% placebo vs. 33% BN52021).

Subsequent studies (n=608) did not confirm any beneficial effect of PAF receptor antagonism on the overall mortality [25]. Controversial results have been obtained from asthmatic patients [19,39] and those suffering from psoriasis [16]. Decreased serum levels of IL-8 and IL-6 were detected after treatment with the PAF antagonist lexipafant in acute human pancreatitis [43].

After the encouraging animal studies with PAF antagonists the few existing clinical trials in fact demonstrated improvement of rheumatic conditions but did not show beneficial effects on survival rates in sepsis. Hence it remains to be elucidated whether or not PAF receptor antagonists can reach significance in the therapy of the critically ill patient.

2.5. References

[1] Ahmad S. N., Alam S. Q., Alam B. S. (1990) Influence of dietary omega-3 fatty acids on transmembrane signalling in rat submandibular salivary gland. *Cell Signal.* 2:29-41.

[2] Allison M. C., Howatson A. G., Torrance C. J., Lee F. D., Russell R. I. (1992) Gastrointestinal damage associated with the use of nonsteroidal antiinflammatory drugs. *N.Engl.J.Med.* 327:749-754.

[3] Arni R. K.Ward R. J. (1996) Phospholipase A2--a structural review. *Toxicon* 34:827-841.

[4] Axelrod L., Camuso J., Williams E., Kleinman K., Briones E., Schoenfeld D. (1994) Effects of a small quantity of omega-3 fatty acids on cardiovascular risk factors in NIDDM. A randomized, prospective, double-blind, controlled study. *Diabetes Care* 17:37-44.

[5] Bernard G. R., Wheeler A. P., Russell J. A., Schein R., Summer W. R., Steinberg K. P., Fulkerson W. J., Wright P. E., Christman B. W., Dupont W. D., Higgins S. B., Swindell B. B. (1997) The effects of ibuprofen on the physiology and survival of patients with sepsis. The Ibuprofen in Sepsis Study Group. *N.Engl.J.Med.* 336:912-918.

[6] Breil I., Koch T., Heller A., Schlotzer E., Grunert A., van Ackern K., Neuhof H. (1996) Alteration of n-3 fatty acid composition in lung tissue after short-term infusion of fish oil emulsion attenuates inflammatory vascular reaction. *Crit Care Med.* 24:1893-1902.

[7] Calder P. C. (2002) Dietary modification of inflammation with lipids. *Proc.Nutr.Soc.* 61:345-358.

[8] Cameron N. E.Cotter M. A. (1993) Potential therapeutic approaches to the treatment or prevention of diabetic neuropathy: evidence from experimental studies. *Diabet.Med.* 10:593-605.

[9] Christman B. W., Lefferts P. L., Blair I. A., Snapper J. R. (1990) Effect of platelet-activating factor receptor antagonism on endotoxin-induced lung dysfunction in awake sheep. *Am.Rev.Respir.Dis.* 142:1272-1278.

[10] de Gomez Dumm, IBrenner R. R. (1975) Oxidative desaturation of alpha-linoleic, linoleic, and stearic acids by human liver microsomes. *Lipids* 10:315-317.

[11] DeCaterina R., Giannessi D., Mazzone A., Bernini W., Lazzerini G., Maffei S., Cerri M., Salvatore L., Weksler B. (1990) Vascular prostacyclin is increased in patients ingesting omega-3 polyunsaturated fatty acids before coronary artery bypass graft surgery. *Circulation* 82:428-438.

[12] Dehmer G. J., Popma J. J., van den Berg E. K., Eichhorn E. J., Prewitt J. B., Campbell W. B., Jennings L., Willerson J. T., Schmitz J. M. (1988) Reduction in the rate of early restenosis after coronary angioplasty by a diet supplemented with n-3 fatty acids. *N.Engl.J.Med.* 319:733-740.

[13] Dhainaut J. F., Tenaillon A., Le Tulzo Y., Schlemmer B., Solet J. P., Wolff M., Holzapfel L., Zeni F., Dreyfuss D., Mira J. P., . (1994) Platelet-activating factor

receptor antagonist BN 52021 in the treatment of severe sepsis: a randomized, double-blind, placebo-controlled, multicenter clinical trial. BN 52021 Sepsis Study Group. *Crit Care Med.* 22:1720-1728.

[14] Diboune M., Ferard G., Ingenbleek Y., Bourguignat A., Spielmann D., Scheppler-Roupert C., Tulasne P. A., Calon B., Hasselmann M., Sauder P., . (1993) Soybean oil, blackcurrant seed oil, medium-chain triglycerides, and plasma phospholipid fatty acids of stressed patients. *Nutrition* 9:344-349.

[15] Dyerberg J., Bang H. O., Hjorne N. (1975) Fatty acid composition of the plasma lipids in Greenland Eskimos. Am.J.Clin.Nutr. 28:958-966.

[16] Elbers M. E., Gerritsen M. J., van de Kerkhof P. C. (1994) The effect of topical application of the platelet-activating factor-antagonist, Ro 24-0238, in psoriasis vulgaris--a clinical and immunohistochemical study. *Clin Exp.Dermatol.* 19:453-457.

[17] Erickson K. L., Hubbard N. E., Chakrabarti R. (1995) Modulation of signal transduction in macrophages by dietary fatty acids. *J.Nutr.* 125:1683S-1686S.

[18] Etienne A., Hecquet F., Soulard C. (1985) In vivo inhibition of plasma protein leakage and Salmonella enterididis-induced mortality in the rat by a specific platelet activating factor acether antagonist BN52021. *Agents Actions* 17:369-370.

[19] Evans D. J., Barnes P. J., Cluzel M., O'Connor B. J. (1997) Effects of a potent platelet-activating factor antagonist, SR27417A, on allergen-induced asthmatic responses. *Am.J.Respir.Crit Care Med.* 156:11-16.

[20] Evans D. J., Barnes P. J., Spaethe S. M., van Alstyne E. L., Mitchell M. I., O'Connor B. J. (1996) Effect of a leukotriene B4 receptor antagonist, LY293111, on allergen induced responses in asthma. *Thorax* 51:1178-1184.

[21] Fearon K. C. H. (2002) The anticancer and anticachectic effects of n-3 fatty acids. *Clin Nutr* 21:69-73.

[22] Fernandes G., Venkatraman J., Khare A., Horbach G. J., Friedrichs W. (1990) Modulation of gene expression in autoimmune disease and aging by food restriction and dietary lipids. *Proc.Soc.Exp.Biol.Med.* 193:16-22.

[23] Fischer S.Weber P. C. (1984) Prostaglandin I3 is formed in vivo in man after dietary eicosapentaenoic acid. *Nature* 307:165-168.

[24] Fox P. L.DiCorleto P. E. (1988) Fish oils inhibit endothelial cell production of platelet-derived growth factor-like protein. *Science* 241:453-456.

[25] Froon A. M., Greve J. W., Buurman W. A., van der Linden C. J., Langemeijer H. J., Ulrich C., Bourgeois M. (1996) Treatment with the platelet-activating factor antagonist TCV-309 in patients with severe systemic inflammatory response syndrome: a prospective, multi-center, double-blind, randomized phase II trial. *Shock* 5:313-319.

[26] Furst D. E. (1997) Meloxicam: selective COX-2 inhibition in clinical practice. *Semin.Arthritis Rheum.* 26:21-27.

[27] Galli C., Trzeciak H. I., Paoletti R. (1971) Effects of dietary fatty acids on the fatty acid composition of brain etanolamine phosphoglyceride. Reciprocal replacement of n-6 and n-3 polyunsaturated fatty acids. *Biochem.Biophys.Acta* 248:449-454.

[28] Gapinski J. P., VanRuiswyk J. V., Heudebert G. R., Schectman G. S. (1993) Preventing restenosis with fish oils following coronary angioplasty. A meta-analysis. *Arch.Intern.Med.* 153:1595-1601.

[29] Glaser K. B., Sung M. L., Hartman D. A., Lock Y. W., Bauer J., Walter T., Carlson R. P. (1995) Cellular and topical in vivo inflammatory murine models in the evaluation of inhibitors of phospholipase A2. *Skin Pharmacol.* 8:300-308.

[30] Goldman D. W., Pickett W. C., Goetzl E. J. (1983) Human neutrophil chemotactic and degranulating activities of leukotriene B5 (LTB5) derived from eicosapentaenoic acid. *Biochem.Biophys.Res.Commun.* 117:282-288.

[31] Grundt H., Nilsen D. W., Hetland O., Aarsland T., Baksaas I., Grande T., Woie L. (1995) Improvement of serum lipids and blood pressure during intervention with n-3 fatty acids was not associated with changes in insulin levels in subjects with combined hyperlipidaemia. *J.Intern.Med.* 237:249-259.

[32] Guth B. D.Muller T. H. (1997) DTTX30, a combined thromboxane receptor antagonist and thromboxane synthetase inhibitor, prevents coronary thrombosis in anesthetized dogs. *Basic Res.Cardiol.* 92:181-190.

[33] Harris R. R., Carter G. W., Bell R. L., Moore J. L., Brooks D. W. (1995) Clinical activity of leukotriene inhibitors. *Int.J.Immunopharmacol.* 17:147-156.

[34] Harris W. S., Windsor S. L., Dujovne C. A. (1991) Effects of four doses of n-3 fatty acids given to hyperlipidemic patients for six months. *J.Am.Coll.Nutr.* 10:220-227.

[35] Heller A., Koch T., Schmeck J., van Ackern K. (1998) Lipid mediators in inflammatory disorders. *Drugs* 55:487-496.

[36] Heller A. R., Theilen H. J., Koch T. (2003) Fish or chips? *News Physiol Sci.* 18:50-54.

[37] Hilliquin P., Guinot P., Chermat-Izard V., Puechal X., Menkes C. J. (1995) Treatment of rheumatoid arthritis with platelet activating factor antagonist BN 50730. *J.Rheumatol.* 22:1651-1654.

[38] Hosford D.Braquet P. (1990) The potential role of platelet activating factor in shock and ischemia. *J.Crit.Care* 5:115-136.

[39] Hozawa S., Haruta Y., Ishioka S., Yamakido M. (1995) Effects of a PAF antagonist, Y-24180, on bronchial hyperresponsiveness in patients with asthma. *Am.J.Respir.Crit Care Med.* 152:1198-1202.

[40] Israel E., Fischer A. R., Rosenberg M. A., Lilly C. M., Callery J. C., Shapiro J., Cohn J., Rubin P., Drazen J. M. (1993) The pivotal role of 5-lipoxygenase products in the reaction of aspirin-sensitive asthmatics to aspirin. *Am.Rev.Respir.Dis.* 148:1447-1451.

[41] Jackson M. D. (1997) Obstuctive airway disease: Unmet needs. Meeting report. *Inflamm.Res.* 46:242-

[42] Kelbel I., Koch T., Prechtl A., Heller A., Schlotzer E., Schiefer G., Neuhof H. (1999) Effects of Parenteral Application of Fish Oil versus Soy Oil Emulsions on Bacterial Clearance functions. *Infusionsther.Transfusionsmed.* 26:226-232.

[43] Kingsnorth A. N., Galloway S. W., Formela L. J. (1995) Randomized, double-blind phase II trial of Lexipafant, a platelet-activating factor antagonist, in human acute pancreatitis. *Br.J.Surg.* 82:1414-1420.

[44] Koch T., Heller A. (2002) Effects of intravenous fish oil on pulmonary integrity and function. *Clin Nutr* 21:41-45.

[45] Koike K., Moore E. E., Moore F. A., Carl V. S., Pitman J. M., Banerjee A. (1992) Phospholipase A2 inhibition decouples lung injury from gut ischemia-reperfusion. *Surgery* 112:173-180.

[46] Kramer R. M.Sharp J. D. (1995) Recent insights into the structure, function and biology of cPLA2. *Agents Actions Suppl* 46:65-76.

[47] Laird J. M., Herrero J. F., Garcia de la Rubia P., Cervero F. (1997) Analgesic activity of the novel COX-2 preferring NSAID, meloxicam in mono-arthritic rats: central and peripheral components. *Inflamm.Res.* 46:203-210.

[48] Landymore R. W., MacAulay M., Sheridan B., Cameron C. (1986) Comparison of cod-liver oil and aspirin-dipyridamole for the prevention of intimal hyperplasia in autologous vein grafts. *Ann.Thorac.Surg.* 41:54-57.

[49] Leaf A. (1990) Cardiovascular effects of fish oils. Beyond the platelet. *Circulation* 82:624-628.

[50] Lee J. Y., Plakidas A., Lee W. H., Heikkinen A., Chanmugam P., Bray G., Hwang D. H. (2003) Differential modulation of Toll-like receptors by fatty acids: preferential inhibition by n-3 polyunsaturated fatty acids. *J.Lipid Res.* 44:479-486.

[51] Lee J. Y., Sohn K. H., Rhee S. H., Hwang D. (2001) Saturated fatty acids, but not unsaturated fatty acids, induce the expression of cyclooxygenase-2 mediated through Toll-like receptor 4. *J.Biol.Chem.* 276:16683-16689.

[52] Lee T. H., Hoover R. L., Williams J. D., Sperling R. I., Ravalese J., III, Spur B. W., Robinson D. R., Corey E. J., Lewis R. A., Austen K. F. (1985) Effect of dietary enrichment with eicosapentaenoic and docosahexaenoic acids on in vitro neutrophil and monocyte leukotriene generation and neutrophil function. *N.Engl.J.Med.* 312:1217-1224.

[53] Lee T. H., Sethi T., Crea A. E., Peters W., Arm J. P., Horton C. E., Walport M. J., Spur B. W. (1988) Characterization of leukotriene B3: comparison of its biological activities with leukotriene B4 and leukotriene B5 in complement receptor enhancement, lysozyme release and chemotaxis of human neutrophils. *Clin.Sci.*(Lond) 74:467-475.

[54] Lewis R. A., Lee T. H., Austen K. F. (1986) Effects of omega-3-fatty acids on the generation of products of the 5-lipoxygenase pathway. In: Simopoulos, A. P. (Hrsg.) Health effects of polyunsaturated fatty acids in seafoods, Academic Press. *Aufl.* 227-238.

[55] Marder P., Spaethe S. M., Froelich L. L., Cerimele B. J., Petersen B. H., Tanner T., Lucas R. A. (1996) Inhibition of ex vivo neutrophil activation by oral LY293111, a novel leukotriene B4 receptor antagonist. *Br.J.Clin Pharmacol.* 42:457-464.

[56] Mayer K., Fegbeutel C., Hattar K., Sibelius U., Kramer H. J., Heuer K. U., Temmesfeld-Wollbruck B., Gokorsch S., Grimminger F., Seeger W. (2003) Omega-3 vs. omega-6 lipid emulsions exert differential influence on neutrophils in septic shock patients: impact on plasma fatty acids and lipid mediator generation. *Intensive Care Med.* 29:1472-1481.

[57] Mensink R. P.Katan M. B. (1990) Effect of dietary trans fatty acids on high-density and low-density lipoprotein cholesterol levels in healthy subjects. *N.Engl.J.Med.* 323:439-445.

[58] Metz C. A.Sheagren J. N. (1990) Ibuprofen in animal models of septic shock. *J.Crit.Care* 5:206-212.

[59] Miguelez R., Palacios I., Navarro F., Gutierrez S., Sanchez-Pernaute O., Egido J., Gonzalez E., Herrero-Beaumont G. (1996) Anti-inflammatory effect of a PAF receptor

antagonist and a new molecule with antiproteinase activity in an experimental model of acute urate crystal arthritis. *J.Lipid Mediat.Cell Signal.* 13:35-49.

[60] Molvig J., Pociot F., Worsaae H., Wogensen L. D., Baek L., Christensen P., Mandrup-Poulsen T., Andersen K., Madsen P., Dyerberg J., . (1991) Dietary supplementation with omega-3-polyunsaturated fatty acids decreases mononuclear cell proliferation and interleukin-1 beta content but not monokine secretion in healthy and insulin-dependent diabetic individuals. *Scand.J.Immunol.* 34:399-410.

[61] Morris M. C. (1994) Dietary fats and blood pressure. *J.Cardiovasc.Risk* 1:21-30.

[62] Morris M. C., Sacks F., Rosner B. (1993) Does fish oil lower blood pressure? A meta-analysis of controlled trials. *Circulation* 88:523-533.

[63] Needleman P., Raz A., Minkes M. S., Ferrendelli J. A., Sprecher H. (1979) Triene prostaglandins: prostacyclin and thromboxane biosynthesis and unique biological properties. *Proc.Natl.Acad.Sci.U.S.A* 76:944-948.

[64] Neuhof H., Seeger W., Suttorp N. (1987) Activation of the pulmonary arachidonic acid system and its consequences for hemodynamics and fluid balance. *Prog.Clin.Biol.Res.* 236A:289-300.

[65] Nickerson-Nutter C. L.Medvedeff E. D. (1996) The effect of leukotriene synthesis inhibitors in models of acute and chronic inflammation. *Arthritis Rheum.* 39:515-521.

[66] Pacht E. R., DeMichele S. J., Nelson J. L., Hart J., Wennberg A. K., Gadek J. E. (2003) Enteral nutrition with eicosapentaenoic acid, gamma-linolenic acid, and antioxidants reduces alveolar inflammatory mediators and protein influx in patients with acute respiratory distress syndrome. *Crit Care Med.* 31:491-500.

[67] Pietsch A., Weber C., Goretzki M., Weber P. C., Lorenz R. L. (1995) N-3 but not N-6 fatty acids reduce the expression of the combined adhesion and scavenger receptor CD36 in human monocytic cells. *Cell Biochem.Funct.* 13:211-216.

[68] Prescott S. M. (1985) The effect of eicosapentaenoic acid on leukotriene B production by human neutrophils. *J.Biol.Chem.* 250:7615-7622.

[69] Pscheidl E., Schywalsky M., Tschaikowsky K., Boke-Prols T. (2000) Fish oil-supplemented parenteral diets normalize splanchnic blood flow and improve killing of translocated bacteria in a low-dose endotoxin rat model. *Crit Care Med.* 28:1489-1496.

[70] Razzini E.Baronzio G. F. (1993) Omega-3 fatty acids as coadjuvant treatment in AIDS. *Med.Hypotheses* 41:300-305.

[71] Rocha F. A., Andrade L. E., Russo M., Jancar S. (1997) PAF modulates eicosanoids and TNF release in immune-complex arthritis in rats. *J.Lipid Mediat.Cell Signal.* 16:1-10.

[72] Sacks F. M., Stone P. H., Gibson C. M., Silverman D. I., Rosner B., Pasternak R. C. (1995) Controlled trial of fish oil for regression of human coronary atherosclerosis. HARP Research Group. *J.Am.Coll.Cardiol.* 25:1492-1498.

[73] Scott K. F., Smith G. M., Green J. A. (1992) Neutralising monoclonal antibody to human secretory phospholipase A2 is anti-hypotensive in a baboon E.coli induced septic shock model. *Prostaglandins and related compounds*

[74] Sebokova E., Garg M. L., Wierzbicki A., Thomson A. B., Clandinin M. T. (1990) Alteration of the lipid composition of rat testicular plasma membranes by dietary (n-3)

fatty acids changes the responsiveness of Leydig cells and testosterone synthesis. *J.Nutr.* 120:610-618.

[75] Seed M. P.Willoughby D. A. (1997) COX-2, HO NO! Cyclooxygenase-2, heme oxygenase and nitric oxide synthase: their role and interactions in inflammation. BIRAs Symposium, Saint Bartholomew's Hospital, London, 26 April 1996. *Inflamm.Res.* 46:279-281.

[76] Seeger W., Wolf H., Stahler G., Neuhof H., Roka L. (1981) [Increase of pulmonary vascular resistance and permeability due to the metabolism of free arachidonic acid (author's transl)]. *Klin.Wochenschr.* 59:459-461.

[77] Sethi S. (2002) Inhibition of leukocyte-endothelial interactions by oxidized omega-3 fatty acids: a novel mechanism for the anti-inflammatory effects of omega-3 fatty acids in fish oil. *Redox.Rep.* 7:369-378.

[78] Sheng G. G., Shao J., Sheng H., Hooton E. B., Isakson P. C., Morrow J. D., Coffey R. J., Jr., DuBois R. N., Beauchamp R. D. (1997) A selective cyclooxygenase 2 inhibitor suppresses the growth of H-ras-transformed rat intestinal epithelial cells. *Gastroenterology* 113:1883-1891.

[79] Sheth K.Bankey P. (2001) The liver as an immune organ. *Curr.Opin.Crit Care* 7:99-104.

[80] Shimokawa H.Vanhoutte P. M. (1988) Dietary cod-liver oil improves endothelium-dependent responses in hypercholesterolemic and atherosclerotic porcine coronary arteries. Circulation 78:1421-1430.

[81] Simopoulos AP, Leaf A, Salem N Jr. Essentiality of and recommended dietary intakes for omega-6 and omega-3 fattyacids.Ann Nutr Metab. 1999;43(2):127-30.

[82] Sperling R. I., Benincaso A. I., Knoell C. T., Larkin J. K., Austen K. F., Robinson D. R. (1993) Dietary omega-3 polyunsaturated fatty acids inhibit phosphoinositide formation and chemotaxis in neutrophils. *J.Clin.Invest* 91:651-660.

[83] Sperling R. I., Robin J. L., Kylander K. A., Lee T. H., Lewis R. A., Austen K. F. (1987) The effects of N-3 polyunsaturated fatty acids on the generation of platelet-activating factor-acether by human monocytes. *J.Immunol.* 139:4186-4191.

[84] Strasser T., Fischer S., Weber P. C. (1985) Leukotriene B5 is formed in human neutrophils after dietary supplementation with icosapentaenoic acid. *Proc.Natl.Acad.Sci.*U.S.A 82:1540-1543.

[85] Taylor I. K., O'Shaughnessy K. M., Fuller R. W., Dollery C. T. (1991) Effect of cysteinyl-leukotriene receptor antagonist ICI 204.219 on allergen-induced bronchoconstriction and airway hyperreactivity in atopic subjects. *Lancet* 337:690-694.

[86] Weber C., Aepfelbacher M., Lux I., Zimmer B., Weber P. C. (1991) Docosahexaenoic acid inhibits PAF and LTD4 stimulated [Ca2+]i-increase in differentiated monocytic U937 cells. *Biochim.Biophys.Acta* 1133:38-45.

[87] Weber P. C. (1990) Fish oil fatty acids and cardiovascular function: epidemiology and biochemical mechanisms. *Biochem.Soc.Trans.* 18:1045-1049.

[88] Weber P. C., Fischer S., von Schacky C., Lorenz R., Strasser T. (1986) Dietary omega-3 polyunsaturated fatty acids and eicosanoid formation in man. In: Simopoulos, A. P. (Hrsg.) Health effects of polyunsaturated fatty acids in seafoods., Academic Press. *Aufl.* 49-60.

[89] Weiner B. H., Ockene I. S., Levine P. H., Cuenoud H. F., Fisher M., Johnson B. F., Daoud A. S., Jarmolych J., Hosmer D., Johnson M. H., . (1986) Inhibition of atherosclerosis by cod-liver oil in a hyperlipidemic swine model. *N.Engl.J.Med.* 315:841-846.

[90] Weinroth S. E., Parenti D. M., Simon G. L. (1995) Wasting syndrome in AIDS: pathophysiologic mechanisms and therapeutic approaches. Infect.Agents Dis. 4:76-94.

[91] Weiss G., Meyer F., Matthies B., Pross M., Koenig W., Lippert H. (2002) Immunomodulation by perioperative administration of n-3 fatty acids. *Br.J.Nutr.* 87 Suppl 1:S89-S94.

[92] Weller P. F., Lee C. W., Foster D. W., Corey E. J., Austen K. F., Lewis R. A. (1983) Generation and metabolism of 5-lipoxygenase pathway leukotrienes by human eosinophils: predominant production of leukotriene C4. *Proc.Natl.Acad.Sci.*U.S.A 80:7626-7630.

[93] Westerveld H. T., de Graaf J. C., van Breugel H. H., Akkerman J. W., Sixma J. J., Erkelens D. W., Banga J. D. (1993) Effects of low-dose EPA-E on glycemic control, lipid profile, lipoprotein(a), platelet aggregation, viscosity, and platelet and vessel wall interaction in NIDDM. *Diabetes Care* 16:683-688.

[94] Wolfram G. (1995) ω-3-Fettsäuren - ihr Stoffwechsel und ihre Wirkungen auf vaskuläres System, Fettstoffwechsel und Immunsystem. *Aktuel.Ernaehr.Med.* 20:179-

[95] Yedgar S., Dan P., Dagan A., Ginsburg I., Lossos I. S., Breuer R. (1995) Control of inflammatory processes by cell-impermeable inhibitors of phospholipase A2. *Agents Actions Suppl* 46:77-84.

[96] Yoshimoto T., Soberman R. J., Lewis R. A., Austen K. F. (1985) Isolation and characterization of leukotriene C4 synthetase of rat basophilic leukemia cells. *Proc.Natl.Acad.Sci.*U.S.A 82:8399-8403.

[97] Zwissler B., Kemming G., Habler O., Kleen M., Merkel M., Haller M., Briegel J., Welte M., Peter K. (1996) Inhaled prostacyclin (PGI2) versus inhaled nitric oxide in adult respiratory distress syndrome. *Am.J.Respir.Crit Care Med.* 154:1671-1677.

[98] Topol EJ (2004) Failing the public health – rofecoxib, Merck, and the FDA. *N Engl J Med* 351:1707–1709

In: Omega 3 Fatty Acids in Clinical Nutrition
Editors: A. Heller, S. Stehr and T. Koch, pp. 29-75
ISBN 1-59454-601-0

Chapter III

Specific Aspects of Omega-3 Fatty Acids

Axel R. Heller and Thea Koch

3.1. Immunological Aspects of Omega-3 Fatty Acids

For a better understanding of the fish oil effects on the complex regulated immunological network the acute phase response is divided into cellular and humoral aspects. The reaction of an immunologically active cell is not dependent on the concentration of one single but rather on a multitude of mediators and receptors as well as on the interaction with various other cells [14]. Thus, therapeutic strategies aiming towards immune-augmentation alone bear the risk of additional tissue damage [123]. Anti-inflammatory interventions on the other hand depress host defense and place the patient at risk of immune compromise [58]. Moreover, monocausal therapeutic interventions regardless of the direction (immuno-stimulating or -depressing) remain without effect [2,27,129,137], considering the immunologic network's transmitting of inflammatory signals occurs simultaneously and redundantly. Further, the up-regulation of surface or cytosolic receptors enables signal transduction despite low signal-density [14].

Through positive feedback loops inflammatory activation in host defense can induce hyper-inflammatory states [34] with subsequent severe tissue injury, culminating in multiple organ failure, in particular, when parallel anti-inflammatory control mechanisms are depressed. Omega-3 FA seem to be capable of lessening hyper-inflammatory processes, by changing cell-to-cell signal transduction [43]. Other features of host defense, however, are enhanced by omega-3 fatty acids without inducing hyper-inflammatory states. Moreover, the post-aggression metabolism was improved. This complex regulation on the one hand brought about by a reduced release of pro-inflammatory arachidonic acid-derivatives and PAF and on the other hand by the amplification of anti-inflammatory EPA-derivatives, which lower the formation of cytokines such as TNF [26,32] and IL-1 [99] in monocytes without inhibiting phagocytosis, burst activity or bactericidal activity of alveolar macrophages [105].

In this context the dynamic course of time of the inflammatory reaction has to be taken into account: the early phase (0-72 h) is characterized by the predominance of pro-inflammatory cytokines TNFα, IL-1, IL-6, IL-8 and the late phase by the predominance of anti-inflammatory cytokines IL-4, IL-10, IL-13 and TGFβ. This course of cytokine production can differ in patients with recurrent septic episodes. Future therapeutical strategies will depend on the prompt determination of the individual immune status and individual genetic disposition. These factors will then determine the interpretation of serum cytokine levels and potential inhibition or augmentation of cytokine cascades.

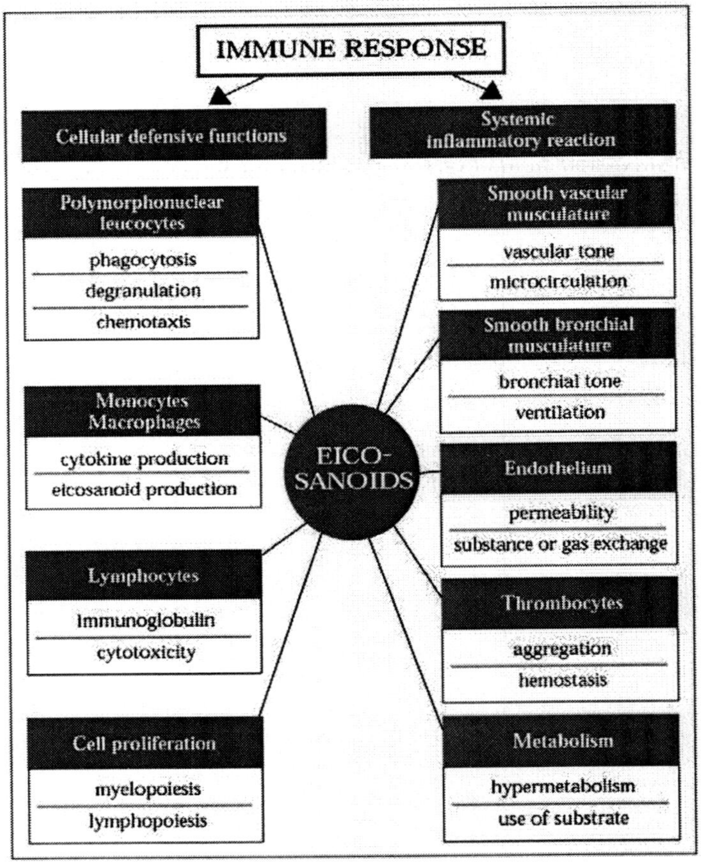

Figure 8. The role of eicosanoids in modulation of the immune response

3.1.1. Effects of Omega-3 FA on the Mononuclear Phagocytosis System

Monocytes and macrophages are immune cells involved in phagocytosis, antigen presentation and cytokine production. Depression of the mononuclear phagocytosis system (MPS) and a dysfunction of the intestinal barrier have been observed after injury or surgical trauma and sepsis. As a consequence large numbers of bacteria and endotoxin enter the bloodstream. The impairment of functions effecting bacterial clearance, caused by reduced phagocytosis and the lysis capability of the MPS is a key issue within the complex pathophysiology of inflammation. Experimental studies regarding the effects of lipid emulsions on phagocytosis by MPS are controversial. Several trials have studied the effects on circulating and resident macrophages in different rodent species. Soy-bean oil enriched parenteral nutrition has been associated with decreased phagocytosis and increased superoxide production by peritoneal macrophages, splenic macrophage proliferation and bacterial translocation [117]. The intravenous infusion in rats infected with *E. coli* resulted in hyperplasia of Kupffer cells and splenic histiocytes [130]. The infusion in guinea pigs reduced the phagocytosis of *E. coli* by Kupffer cells and splenic macrophages [50].

Control of eicosanoid synthesis attenuates overwhelming inflammatory reactions which ultimately may lead to organ failure [55,61]. However, intact generation of eicosanoid and proper regulation of their production is of major importance for maintaining a systemic and cellular host defense. A series of functional alterations induced by diets enriched with omega-3 FA might contribute to the described effects, i.e. an increased production of cytokines, increases of cell-mediated immunity and opsonisation index [4], as well as an increase of antigen-induced lymphocyte generation [23,130]. In animal experiments, Ertel et al. observed an increased cytokine production (Il-1, IL-2), a reduced PGE_2 release from macrophages and an improvement in both the capacity of antigen presentation and splenocyte proliferation following hemorrhagic shock in animals which had been fed omega-3 FA instead of omega -6 FA [33]. Hence, mortality was significantly reduced using diets supplemented with omega-3 FA in animal models of sepsis [11]. The idea that the cellular and humoral defense might be impaired under preferential omega-6 FA application has been supported by in vitro experiments demonstrating that omega -6 FA supplementation results in reduced phagocytosis activity and mitogen-induced proliferation of lymphocytes as well as suppressed synthesis of immunoglobins [75]. Based on these and other observations, appropriate nutritional support with lipid emulsion containing omega-3 FA may ameliorate impaired immune functions after injury, thus reducing the risk of sepsis. Even under conditions of severe illness omega -3 FA reduced the severity of the systemic inflammatory response to infection [61,80], improved patient condition and prolonged survival [107].

We addressed the key question whether omega-3 FA influence phagocytosis and lysis capacity of the MPS and thereby reduce bacterial growth in blood and tissue [73]. In a rabbit bacteremia model we chose a quantitative intravenous administration of *E. coli* as a correlate of bacterial invasion into the circulating blood from various origins, e.g. the gut, the urogenital tract, wounds or implanted catheters.

As opposed to soy oil emulsion, supplementation with omega-3 FA improved MPS phagocytosis, as shown by an enhanced bacterial clearance from the blood and a significantly lower number of bacteria in the lung. The decreased amount of bacteria in the lung in the animals treated with omega-3 FA can be attributed to a reduced lung neutrophil recruitment under improved bacterial clearance conditions on the grounds of reduced leukocyte/ endothelium interaction by lower adhesion molecule expression [85,94]. Moreover, omega-3 FA augment phagocytic cell function through changes in membrane phospholipid content and reduced production of PGE_2 and LTB_4.

Omega-3 EPA competes with the PGE_2 precursor arachidonic acid for binding at the active site of cyclooxygenase, thus resulting in a reduced production of PGE_2, which is one key mediator of immuno-suppression following major injury.

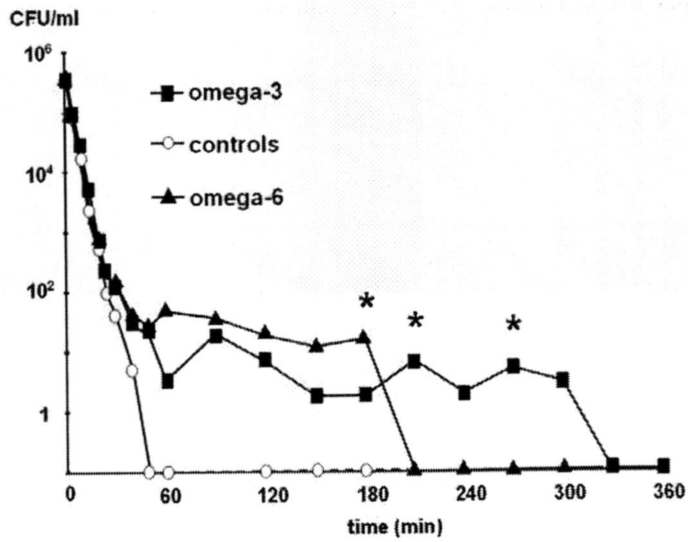

Figure 9. Viable bacteria counts per ml of blood over an observation period of 360 min after injection of *E:coli* ($1.3x10^8$ CFU) in controls animals or animals treated with fish oil or soy bean oil emulsion at a dose of 1.5g/kg/BW for 3 days [73]. (Reprinted with permission of S. Karger AG Medical and Scientific Publishers, Basel, Switzerland, from Kelbel I, et al., Infusionsther. Transfusionsmed. 1999)

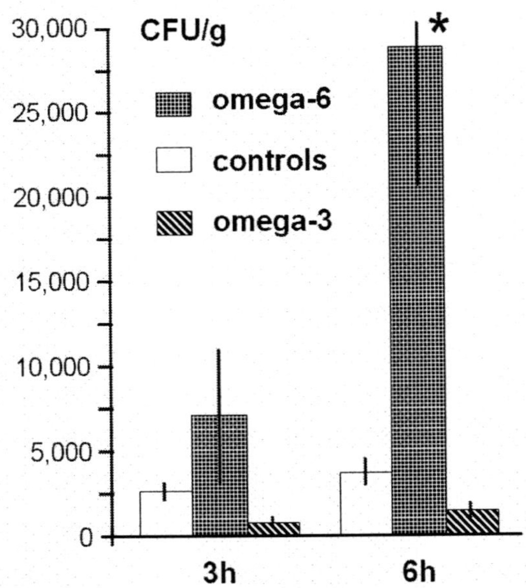

Figure 10. Viable bacteria counts per gram of lung tissue at 3 and 6h after injection of *E:coli* in controls animals or animals treated with fish oil or soy bean oil emulsion at a dose of 1.5g/kg/BW for 3 days [73]. (Reprinted with permission of S. Karger AG Medical and Scientific Publishers, Basel, Switzerland, from Kelbel I, et al., Infusionsther. Transfusionsmed. 1999)

Recent studies have shown that PGE_2 suppresses various aspects of the immune response, including lymphocyte proliferation, lymphokine secretion, and phagocyte function [5,31]. The same applies for LTB_4 which is a chemotactic key mediator.

Further, the effects of enhanced membrane fluidity on phagocyte function by fish oil seem to be a relevant mechanism. Mahoney and coworkers calculated that, under normal conditions, the phagocytosis of an erythrocyte results in an internalization of approximately 7% of the macrophage surface area [89]. Thus, expansion of membrane fluidity by altering the membrane fatty acid composition should facilitate phagocytosis of bacteria.

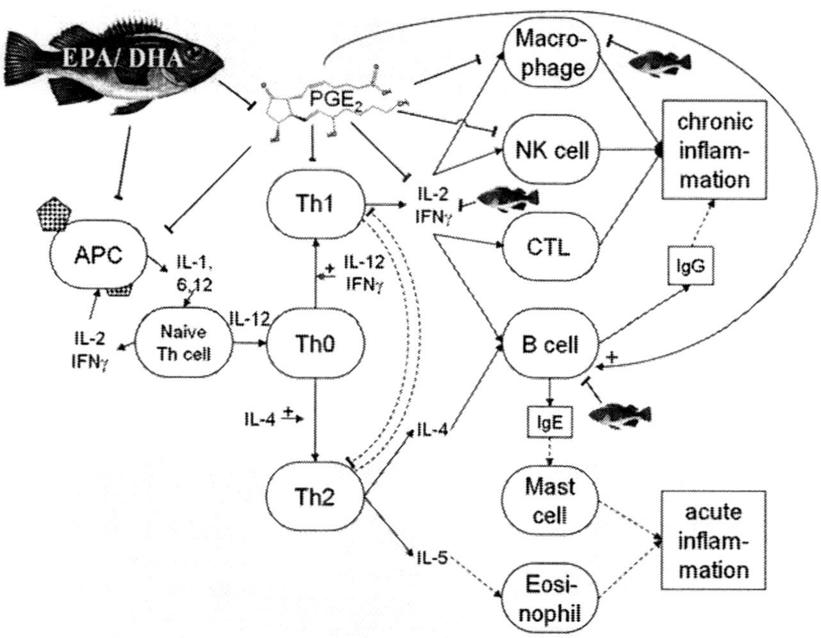

Figure 11. Lymphocytes can be classified as either T or B lymphocytes by the presence of CD3 or CD19, respectively, on their surface. When T lymphocytes are presented with antigen by antigen presenting cells (APC), they become activated, secrete cytokines and ultimately enter the cell cycle and divide. This so-called proliferation of lymphocytes increases the number of antigen-specific lymphocytes and represents the memory of the cell-mediated immune response. T lymphocytes are classified into helper T (Th) cells, distinguished by the presence of the molecule CD4 on their surface and cytotoxic T lymphocytes CTL, presenting CD8 on their surface. Th lymphocytes can be further subdivided according to the expression of CD45 isoforms on their cell surface. It is believed that naive Th cells (i.e., those that have not yet encountered an activating stimulus) express CD45RA, whereas memory Th cells (i.e., those that have been produced as a consequence of exposure to an activating stimulus) express CD45RO. Both Th and Tc lymphocytes can also be subdivided functionally according to the pattern of cytokines that they produce. Type-1 helper or cytotoxic T lymphocytes produce interleukin (IL)-2 and interferon- gamma (IFNγ), whereas type-2 helper or cytotoxic T lymphocytes produce IL-4, IL-5 and IL-10, although T cells are not the only sources of these cytokines [100].

Lymphocytes are poor sources of eicosanoids, even though they are subject to eicosanoids regulation. PGE_2 inhibits lymphocyte proliferation, NK cell activity and the production of Th1 cytokines (IL-2, IFNγ) [75]. PGE_2 also inhibits MHC II expression and the production of TNF-α and IL-1β by monocytes and macrophages. In contrast, PGE_2 does not directly influence IL-4 levels and promotes IgE production by B-lymphocytes [75]. LTB_4 enhances production of TNF-α, IL-1 and IL-6 by monocytes and macrophages as well as enhances Th1 cytokine production and NK cell activity.

Fish oil as a PGE_2 antagonist should increase the production of Th1-type cytokines, enhance MHC II expression, lymphocyte proliferation and NK cell activity, and decrease IgE production by B-lymphocytes. Despite the logic behind these observations some experiments, however, demonstrated effects that are opposed to those predicted on the basis of sole PGE_2 antagonism. Therefore, fish oil is not just a PGE_2 antagonist, but effects seem to be more complex.

Dietary fish oil decreases the graft versus host responses compared with low fat diets or those rich in omega-6 FA or olive oil. Furthermore, dietary fish oil prolongs the survival of skin, kidney, heart or Langerhans islets transplants in rodents [21,22,42,43]. Regarding these results, fish oil seems to induce a shift in the T-lymphocyte response away from the Th1-type response, which is involved in cell-mediated immunity, chronic inflammation and graft rejection.

3.1.2. Impact of Omega-3 FA on Cellular Immune Response in Humans

Human clinical studies investigating the effects of lipid emulsions on leukocyte function are rare. In the past decade initial studies describing the beneficial effects of FO on the regulation of the cellular immune response were performed in chronic inflammatory diseases or autoimmune processes, such as ulcerative colitis [44], atopic dermatitis [95], or rheumatoid arthritis [40]. Interestingly enough, these works focused on diseases in which the imbalance of pro- and anti- inflammatory features is an integral part of the respective pathomechanisms [88]. The observed clinical effects have been explained on the mechanistic grounds of prostanoid and leukotriene antagonism. Clinical parameters such as morning stiffness or joint pain improved after daily doses of 2.6-8g fish oil. Doses of non steroidal antiphlogistics could be reduced or even abandoned [40,82]. Animal studies also revealed that fish oil has beneficial effects on nephritis, induced by lupus erythematosus. Proteinuria and histologic changes were markedly reduced after omega-3 FA diet [110]. Exemplified in acute, extended guttate psoriasis, an inflammatory skin disease characterized by a dysfunction of neutrophils and lymphocytes generating increased levels of pro-inflammatory lipid mediators and cytokines [19], Grimminger and coworkers showed a rapid improvement of clinical manifestations and changes in neutrophil leukotriene profile, lowered neutrophil infiltration and desquamation, as well as advances of the subjective patient assessment after the intravenous application of 2.1g EPA and 21.0g DHA per day [47]. These authors, likewise, demonstrated beneficial effects of 4.2g EPA + 4.2g DHA/d on the course of the disease in a patient with severe ulcerative colitis [44].

In a study conducted by our group, effects of omega-3 FA on the acute phase response were characterized [57]. Major surgical trauma results in a marked elevation of almost all leukocyte populations in the observed cohort of 44 patients (table 7).

Table 7. Effects of major surgical trauma in 44 patients and differential omega fatty acid supplementation for 5 days on leukocyte subpopulations mean±SD *p<0.05 [57]

	Cell counts in relation to major surgery [Pt μl^{-1}]			
	before surgery	**after surgery**	**after surgery and 5 days Omega-6**	**after surgery and 5 days Omega-3**
White blood cells	6,500±4,000	12,600±4,700*	11,400±4,900	12,000±5,900
Neutrophils	3,770±650	10,458 ±1,260*	7,638±912	8,880±1,200
Monocytes (CD14+)	538±323	711±491	1.192±902	975±749
activ. Monocytes (CD14+HLADR+)	382±253	237±242*	697±688	541±361
B-Lymphocytes (CD19+)	194±134	388±1,264	375±633	214±283
T- Lymphocytes (CD3+)	1,161±596	743±474*	1,105±623	963±645
activated T- cells (CD3+HLADR+)	57±50	50±48*	67±66	47±41
T helper cells (CD3+4+)	746±427	446±318*	729±419	674±509
T suppressor cells (CD3+8+)	407±280	279±237*	365±342	291±200
CD4/CD8 ratio	2.24±1.35	2.05±1.41*	2.82±1.65	2.63±1.71
Natural killer cells (CD56+3-)	203±180	188±265	229±202	129±82
Cytolytic T cells (CD56+3+)	45±72	37±45*	39±30	43±54

Increased neutrophil and monocyte counts contributed to leukocytosis on the first postoperative day. The fraction of activated monocytes, however, was cut in half. Interestingly, the fraction of antigen presenting monocytes decreased, as well as the number of T-lymphocytes, their activation level and counts of natural killer cells. Because the decrease of helper T-cells (CD3+4+) was more pronounced than the T-suppressor cell counts (CD3+8+), the pro-inflammatory character of the balance between these two cell types was reduced on the first post-operative day.

Similar results were found by Menges and coworkers following multiple trauma [7]. They observed reduced counts of total lymphocytes, of natural killer cells as well as of CD4+ T-lymphocytes. Accordingly CD4/CD8 ratio dropped. Whether the decrease of immunologically active circulating cells is a result of an enhanced sequestration within the framework of host defense or is due to an emigration of monocytes into organs of the MPS and subsequent transformation into tissue macrophages, is a question that currently can not be answered. A reinforced phagocytosis-function of Kupffer-cells in the liver after hemorrhagic shock [68], however, could point towards an enhanced emigration of circulating immunologically active monocytes into MPS-organs. While natural killer cells (CD56+3-) remain unchanged, cytolytic T-cells (CD56+3+) significantly dropped. Omega-3 FA-supplemented TPN increased neutrophil counts but reduced the number of circulating monocytes.

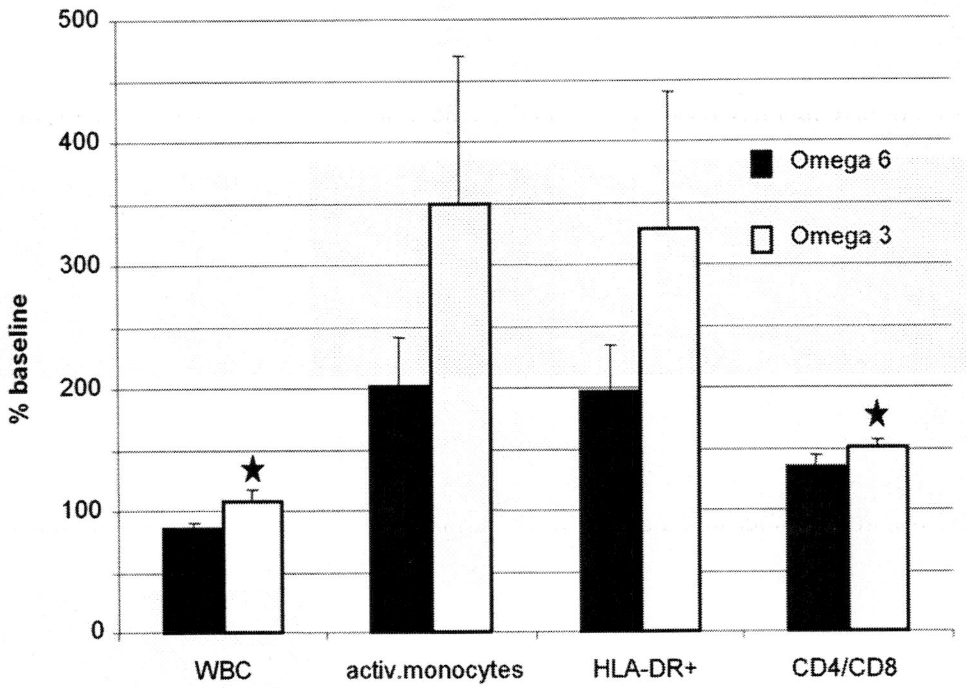

Figure 12. Impact of fish oil supplementation on the cellular immunity of patients after major abdominal surgery and 5 days of parenteral nutrition including fish oil n=24 or soy bean oil n=20

The immuno- stimulating effect of omega-3 FA resulted in a simultaneous increase of cytolytic T-lymphocytes (CD56+3+), of antigen presenting T-lymphocytes (CD3+HLADR+) and of B-lymphocytes. The total number of HLA-DR-positive cells varied considerably from one subject to another and higher mean numbers in the omega-3 group failed to reach statistical significance. Weiss and colleagues were, however, able to detect a preservation of HLA-DR- positive cells [133] in postoperative patients receiving fish oil as opposed to soy bean oil. In the omega-6 group HLA-DR- positive cells significantly dropped. In this regard, omega-3 FA seem to preserve the cellular compensatory potential which is required to balance immune response [54].

Causes for the increase of CTL-counts under supplementation of FO could accordingly be found in an improved activation, proliferation or differentiation of memory T-cells and an enhanced antigen presentation by antigen presenting cells [135].

One anti- inflammatory, immunomodulatory aspect provided by the application of omega-3 FA was a reduction of the number of natural killer cells (CD56+3-), in particular in patients with elevated total white blood cell counts. Considering the results of Tanigushi and co-workers, who observed reduced mortality rates in SIRS patients with lower IL-6/IL-10 ratios [121], it can be postulated that omega-3 FA may have favorable effects under conditions of an overwhelming pro- inflammatory reaction. This hypothesis is supported by the findings that cytolytic T-lymphocytes (CD3+56+) as well as natural killer cells (CD3-56+) showed spontaneous non-MHC-restricted and therefore uncontrolled cytotoxic activity towards a multiplicity of cell types [83]. Further, the potential of omega 3 FA to reduce mortality was the higher, the more organs failed [61]. Although different effects of each of these two potentially competing cell-populations are known, definite and clinically relevant conclusions can up to now not be drawn concerning their interactions or synergisms [83]. Therefore, assumptions regarding the therapeutic value of the opposite regulation of these two cell types under FO-supplementation remain speculative.

Most recently, data on the disease severity related impact of lipid emulsions on phagocyte functions in postoperative as well as in septic patients were provided by Weiss [133] and Mayer [91]. While the differential effects of soy bean oil and fish oil on phagocytosis activity and respiratory burst of phagocytes were not detectable in postoperative patients [133], Mayer and colleagues impressively demonstrated the impact of the type of fatty acid on phagocyte functions when the severity of the illness increases [91]. This group observed a significant depression of oxygen radical production in neutrophils after omega-6 FA [91] as opposed to omega-3 FA. Moreover, they presented data on monocytes of septic patients showing reduced levels of TNF alpha, IL-1, IL-6, and IL-8 due to fish oil administration without affecting the anti-inflammatory IL-10 response [92]. Further, they demonstrated anti- inflammatory effects of fish oil by showing that endothelial monocyte rolling was induced by soy bean oil but not by fish oil, and omega-3 FA significantly reduced adherence and transmigration of monocytes [94]. These results are in line with preliminary data of two clinical trials in which fish oil diets were shown to have restorative effects on the depressed cellular immunity and to improve the condition and survival of patients on intensive care units [74], in particular in progressive states [61].

Altogether the phagocytic response is one of the most complex regulated systems within the mammalian organism. Multitudes of back coupling mechanisms are responsible for up-regulating the immune response and for the subsequent shutdown of hostile responses during recovery. Multiple anti-inflammatory strategies developed over recent decades to cure sepsis have failed. Lessons learned from those studies are that the regulatory complexity of host defense cannot be modulated by one simple anti-inflammatory approach, which on the one hand may save the organism from self-destruction but on the other hand leads to further septic complications. Within this framework omega-3 FA seem to fulfill the role of modulators rather than the part of any pro- or anti-inflammatory player. It is just this fine balance of avoiding both overwhelming inflammation and immuno-paralysis, which must be re-established to enable restoration of homeostasis and recovery. Through a stimulating effect on both the pro- and the anti-inflammatory players, omega-3 FA might serve to offset imbalances of the cellular immune response and, thus, enable rapid restoration of homeostasis and recovery.

3.1.3. Acute Inflammatory Reaction, Humoral Factors, and Omega-3 Fatty Acids

In animal sepsis studies using a cecal ligation model survival was significantly improved after fish oil application [71]. Results from first clinical studies show that the *ex vivo* stimulation of granulocytes in patients receiving fish oil has a lipid mediator spectrum matching omega-3 FA derived mediators [92]. Subsequently, a reduction of several pro-inflammatory cytokines could be observed in the patients' serum [46]. The beneficial pulmonary effects observed *ex vivo* by our group [79,81] were confirmed by the „Enteral Nutrition in ARDS Study Group" in 146 patients with ARDS [38]. An improved gas exchange with a significantly augmented oxygenation index and reduced F_iO_2- und PEEP-levels could be achieved in patients treated with fish oil. Weaning times and ICU dismissal was significantly shortened by fish oil application. Re- evaluation of the patients' serum from this study revealed reduced humoral host response in terms of IL-6, IL-8, TNFα, and LTB_4 and gave the biochemical and pathophysiological rationale for the observed clinical improvement of the patient' condition [104].

Our own group was able to document beneficial effects on the liver itself and a positive hepatic acute phase response in 44 patients after major abdominal surgery (SAPS II 17±6) receiving 0.2g/kg/d fish oil [57]. The effects of surgical trauma on circulatory immunocompetent cells also affected the serum-levels of cytokines and acute-phase proteins. While CRP, interleukin-10 and phospholipase A_2 increased tenfold postoperatively, in comparison to baseline, interleukin-6 reached 100-fold higher values. Accordingly, the pro-/anti-inflammatory balance between IL-6 and IL-10 was significantly postponed in favor of pro-inflammatory IL-6.

The effects of administering fish oil were evident within 24 h. Similar results have been published by Hwang et al. in an animal model of sepsis, showing that ASAT and ALAT as well as mortality and hepatocellular apoptosis were reduced after omega-3 FA application [69]. Our data on improved liver function (see chapter 3.4) are in line with those collected by Pscheidl, who found an improved splanchnic perfusion and reduced bacterial translocation with omega-3 FA [108]. The extension of the "positive hepatic acute phase response" [115] as part of an immuno-stimulant omega-3 FA effect was indicated by increased CRP and fibrinogen levels, the significant increase in neutrophil counts and the relation of helper T-cells to suppressor T-cells. This immune-augmentation could, in part be the result of the improved liver-function, which was reflected by lower transaminases, bilirubin, lactatdehydrogenase, and improved VLDL levels. The stronger hepatic production of proteins of humoral host defense or of coagulation factors [115] correlates with a tendency to higher serum-levels of opsonizing CRP or fibrinogen. Conversely, a weakened acute-phase reaction after burn injury was associated with elevated mortality rates [18]. Omega-3 FA have evened out pro- and anti-inflammatory immunomodulatory effects in a postoperative situation which is dominated by a pro-inflammatory systemic response

On the other hand, anti-inflammatory effects were observed. While the absolute values of IL-6 and IL-10 were the same in controls and omega-3 FA patients, the ratio of IL-6/ IL-10, which was shown to be correlated with mortality in sepsis [121], was cut in half after FO-administration. The 30% increase of PLA_2 concentrations in the omega-6 group on day 3 was found this difference was not statistically significant.

Clinical effects of the optimized acute phase response after omega-3 FA were evident in distinct organ systems even in non-septic postoperative patients. They mainly reflect the organism's lower tendency to edema formation and improved performance of hepatic protein synthesis. This tendency to a lower edema formation on the one hand, and improved postoperative anabolism on the other hand was evident in a weight loss of 1.1 kg in the omega-6 FA group which was absent in the omega-3 FA group despite a 0.5 l lower cumulative ICU fluid-balance after omega-3 FA. Similar improvements of the nutritional state in cancer patients receiving omega-3 FA were reported by Barber [8].

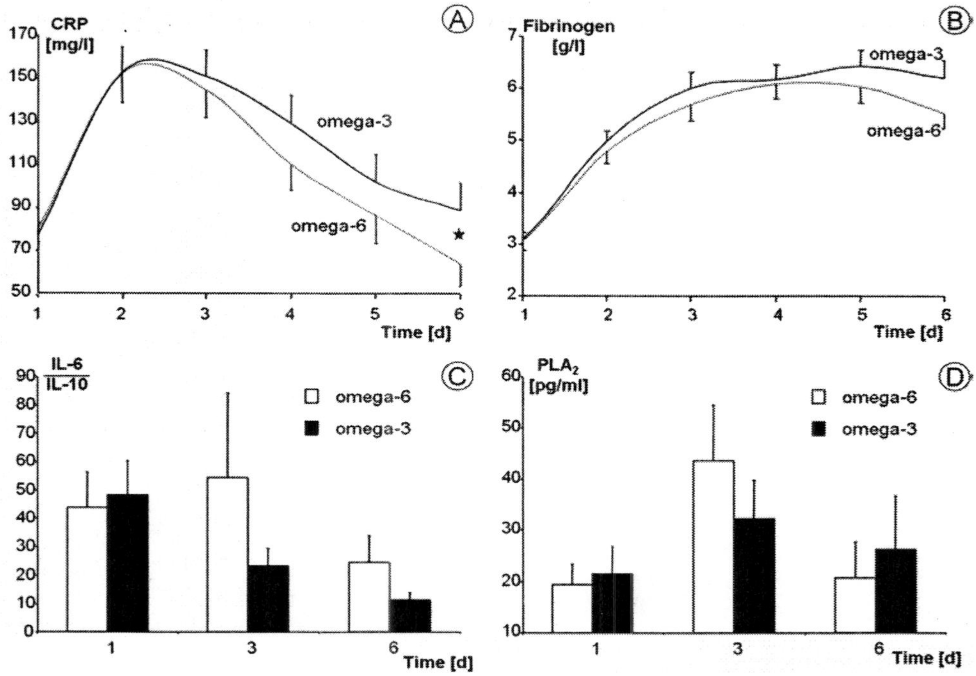

Figure 13. Time course of C- reactive protein CRP (A), fibrinogen (B), IL-6/IL-10 ratio (C), and phospholipase (PLA) A_2 (D) during five day parenteral nutrition with soy oil emulsion or fish oil after major abdominal surgery. (mean±SEM)

Table 8. Acute phase parameters reflecting the pro-/ anti- inflammatory balance of humoral mediators in 44 patients after major abdominal surgery and postoperative with fish oil or soy bean oil.

	Baseline		day 6	
	Omega-6	Omega-3	Omega-6	Omega-3
Body temperature [°C]	37,0±0,4	37,0±0,6	36,5±0,4	36,6±0,5
WBC [GPt l^{-1}]	13,6±4,6	11,9±4,8	11,4±4,9	12,0±5,9
CRP [mg l^{-1}]	9,2±13,1	8,8±10,4	63,6±46,9	88,7±64,3
Fibrinogen [g/l]	3,1±0,7	3,1±0,7	5,5±1,3	6,2±1,7
Procalcitonin [ng ml^{-1}]	0,8±0,7	0,8±0,9	0,2±0,6	0,2±0,2
Interleukin-6 [pg ml^{-1}]	343±464	138±138	44±57	36±50
Interleukin-10 [pg ml^{-1}]	17±18	13±14	6±13	6±7
IL-6/IL-10 Ratio	44±54	48±58	25±39	12±12
Phospholipase A_2 [pg ml^{-1}]	19±18	22±26	21±31	26±51
TNFα and IL-1β	not detected	n.d.	n.d.	n.d.

Postoperatively, the oxygenation-index was significantly depressed in all patients and PaO_2/FiO_2 ratios above 300 mmHg were not regained until day 3. Albeit, a decreased pulmonary edema formation [79] by reduction of capillary leakage [81], which has been reported previously in 146 ARDS patients [38] was expected after omega-3 FA in our postoperative patients, the oxygenation index gave no indication of additional protective effects of omega-3 FA on pulmonary function. The failure to detect differences in the oxygenation index among the groups is very likely due to the fact that postoperative patients in this study fortunately were in a good pulmonary condition.

Taken together, all the described small single improvements of the immunologic balance after omega-3 supplementation allow a faster achievement of homeostasis and consequently a shorter requirement of intensive care, in particular in patients at risk for sepsis with an IL-6/IL-10 ratio of ≥8.

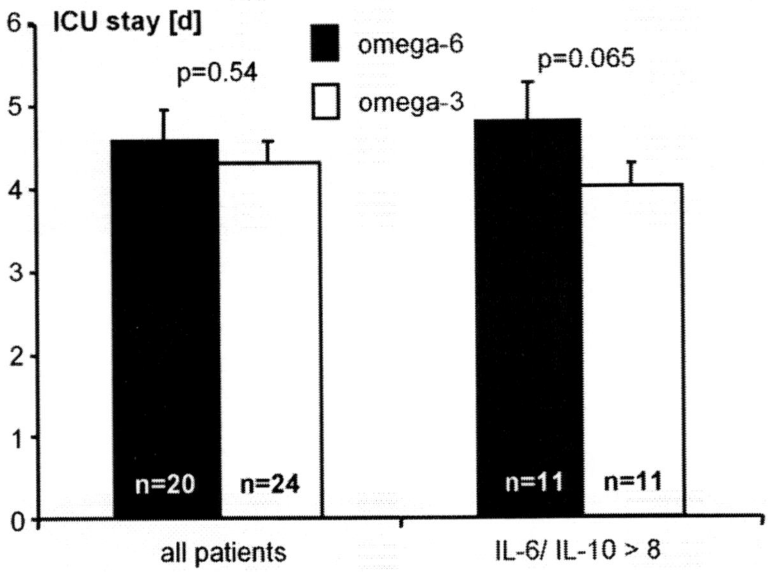

Figure 14. Length of ICU stay in patients after major abdominal surgery and postoperative parenteral nutrition under supplementation with fish oil or soy bean oil. The ratio of IL-6/IL-8 selects patients at risk for sepsis. (Reprinted with permission, International Journal of Cancer © copyright (2004) Wiley-Liss Inc., from Heller AR, et al.)

Supplementation with omega-3 FA has rapid onset immuno-modulatory effects in patients after major abdominal surgery as well as in critically ill patients. The observed modulation is characterized by a certain constellation of immuno-competent cells and their respective cytokines. However, omega-3 FA-effects cannot unequivocally be assigned to the pro- or anti-inflammatory category. Despite the emphasis on the pro-inflammatory aspect in the observed mixed antagonistic reaction (MARS) after major abdominal surgery [17], this condition was classified as a compensated physiological post-aggression metabolism regarding the favorable course of infection parameters as well as the development of SAPS II, procalcitonin levels, and the TNFα and interleukin-1β concentrations below limits of detection.

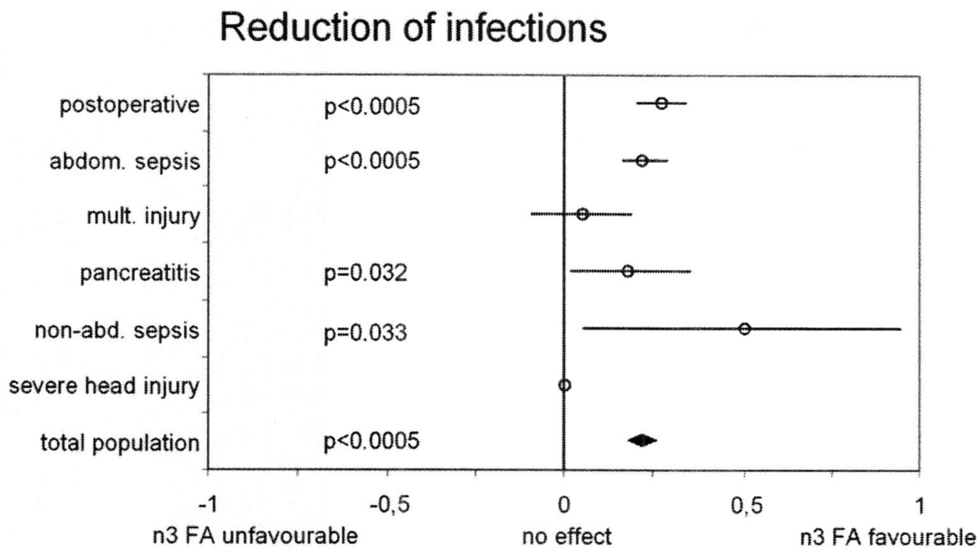

Figure 15. Effects of parenteral administration of omega-3 fatty acids on infection rates from a multicenter study including 661 patients

As a result, the complex actions of omega-3 fatty acids on cellular and humoral host defense induce beneficial clinical effects such as lower infection rates as documented in recent studies investigating various degrees of disease severity [41,74,125]. For a beneficial modulation of immunological imbalances it appears essential to use substances such as fish oil which do not aim towards one single target with a defined pro- or anti- inflammatory intention. Keeping in mind that therapies which are based on immuno-stimulants alone, are associated with the danger of additional tissue-damage [123], and that on the other hand, anti-inflammatory interventions may negatively influence host defense, omega-3 FA could improve host defense without inducing hyper-inflammatory states as well as the post-aggression metabolism through balanced pro- and anti-inflammatory effects on a variety of host defense subsystems. This may in particular apply to patients at risk for sepsis.

3.2. Omega 3 Fatty Acids as Adjunctive in Cancer Patients

Epidemiological studies have indicated that a high intake of saturated fat and/or animal fat increases the risk of colon and breast cancer. Certain polyunsaturated fatty acids contained in fish oil, on the other hand, can inhibit the growth of a variety of human cancer cell lines in vitro [36]. Diets rich in omega-3 FA were claimed to reduce the risk of several types of cancer, including prostate, colorectal, breast [25]. However, a meta-analysis over 38 prospective high quality cancer incidence studies found large hetrogenity between the reported outcomes. The authors concluded that little evidence exists to support omega-3 fatty acid intake to reduce the risk of cancer incidence within a population [51]. While it is difficult to demonstrate prophylactic effects in large populations, therapeutic effects were reported by different groups [9,10,25,36,36]. The mechanisms discussed in the prevention of tumor expansion may also apply to metastatic or residual cancer cells. Thus, consuming omega-3 FA offers a non-toxic way to augment cancer therapy, support chemotherapy and to significantly increase life span.

COX II is increased in a variety of human cancers, including those of the colon, breast, oesophagus, liver, cervix, bladder, and pancreas and may suppress apoptosis. Observations that the inhibition of COX II by NSAIDs prevents tumor growth [127], further support the concept of omega-3 FA administration. Omega-3 FA downregulate COX II- expression, alter its metabolites, and, consequently, avoid the PGE_2 induced increase of estrogen in breast cancer and of a PGH_2- induced further DNA- damage (figure 16). Those pathways have comparable metabolic endpoints as COX II inhibition by NSAIDs. Like all growth processes, cancer growth too is dependent on substrates and therefore on angiogenesis. Vascular endothelial growth factors promoting tumor angiogenesis, however, are favoured by omega-6 FA metabolites such as PGE_2. Omega 3 derivatives do not support VEGF release by PGE_2.

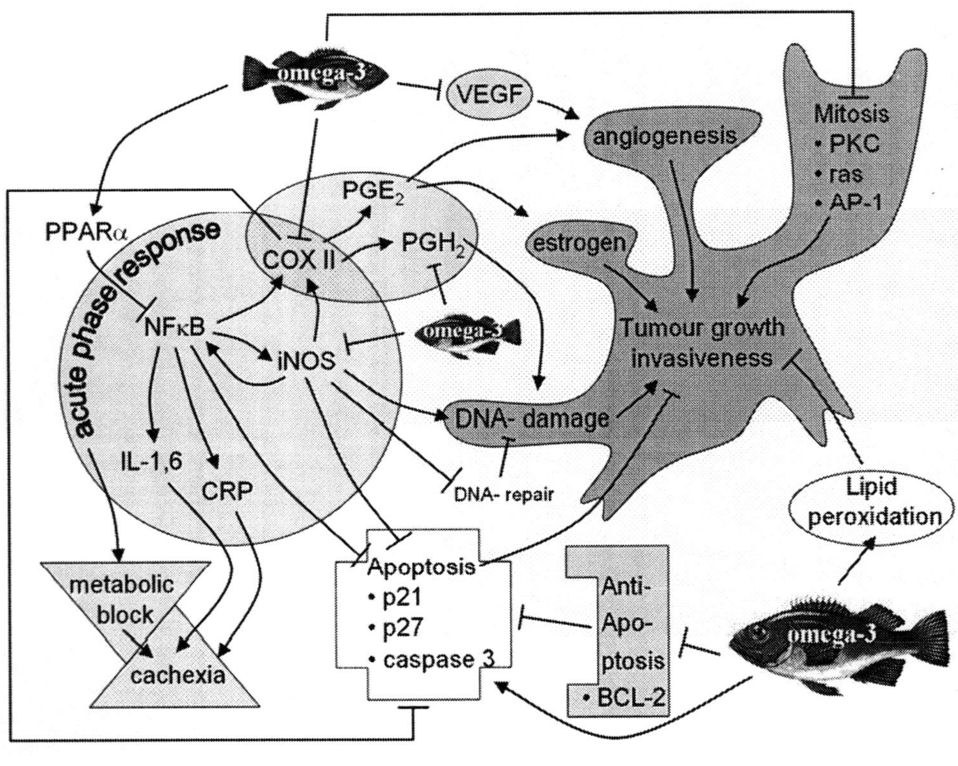

Figure 16. Mechanisms of omega-3 FA action in tumor growth. Cyclooxygenase (COX) II and inducible NO synthase (iNOS) are key propagators of tumor development and inhibitors of tumoricidal activity. →favours activity; ⊥ blocks activity

Inducible NO synthase is another central source of pro- inflammatory and carcinogenic signals and may potentiate inflammation as well as tumor growth, due to its various interfaces to other cascade systems, such as COX and nuclear factor (NF) κB [102]. In avoiding the up-regulation of iNOS by omega-3 FA an excessive secondary activation of mediator systems can be controlled.

Regarding the nuclear key pro-inflammatory transcription factor, NFκB, EPA increases the activity of peroxisome proliferator activated receptors (PPAR), which inhibit the transcriptional activity of NFκB, and therefore regulate tumor promoting hyper-inflammatory activity. Moreover, it is suggested, that EPA might stabilize the NFκB / IκB- complex in the cytoplasm and, consequently, may influence pro- inflammatory cytokine production and inflammatory response [36,112]. In addition, NFκB activation may block apoptotic pathways. By inhibiting NFκB or anti-apoptotic genes such as *BCL-2*, omega-3 FA may conserve tumor destructing apoptotic mechanisms of the host and, therefore, may improve tumor defense.

Further laboratory experiments showed a reduced risk of chemically induced colon carcinogenesis after omega-3 FA. In a phase II clinical trial of patients with colonic polyps, dietary fish oil supplements have inhibited cell proliferation. Mechanisms responsible for anti-tumor effects in animal models include reduced levels of PGE_2, inducible NO synthase as well as an increased lipid peroxidation, or translation inhibition and subsequent cell cycle arrest [36]. While arachidonic acid omega-6 derivatives increase mitosis and therefore may promote tumor growth, omega-3 FA lower the mitosis stimulating proteinkinase C and decrease the activity of the oncogenes *ras* and AP-1. Likewise, dietary fish oil decreased the concentration of secondary bile acids, which act as colon tumor promoters.

Whitehouse provides further molecular insights into the mechanisms of EPA derived prevention of tumor growth [134]. Soleus muscles in mice carrying a cachexia-inducing tumor (MAC16) showed increased protein degradation in vitro. EPA suppressed catabolism through inhibition of an ATP-dependent proteolytic pathway. Proteasome activity was completely suppressed, together with an attenuation of the expression of 20S proteasome alpha-subunits and the p42 regulator, suggesting that EPA induces the attenuation of the up-regulation of proteasome expression in cachectic mice, and this correlated with an increase in skeletal muscle protein expression.

Besides the invasive or non- invasive tumor growth itself, weight loss is a major cause of morbidity and mortality in patients with advanced cancer. While it is possible to increase energy and protein intake enterally or parenterally, this seems to have little impact on the patient's progressive weight loss. This has led to the suggestion that there is a partial metabolic block to the accretion of lean tissue in patients with cancer [98], which may be due to pro-inflammatory cytokines, alterations in the balance of neuroendocrine hormones, and specific, tumor-derived proteolytic and lipid-mobilizing factors. Several clinical studies of recent years provide evidence for beneficial effects of fish oil administration in cancer cachexia and during radio- and chemotherapy. It has been suggested that omega-3 eicosapentaenoic acid (EPA) is capable of down-regulating the production and action of a number of mediators of cachexia, such as IL-1, IL-6, TNFα and proteolysis-inducing factor [112,124]. On the other hand emulsions of soybean oil seem to impede tumoricidal activity as compared to EPA [131]. Barber and co-workers have recently shown that a fish-oil-enriched nutritional supplement reverses weight loss in cachectic cancer patients [10]. Patients suffering from tumor cachexia in pancreatic cancer received a daily dose of 1.1 g EPA.

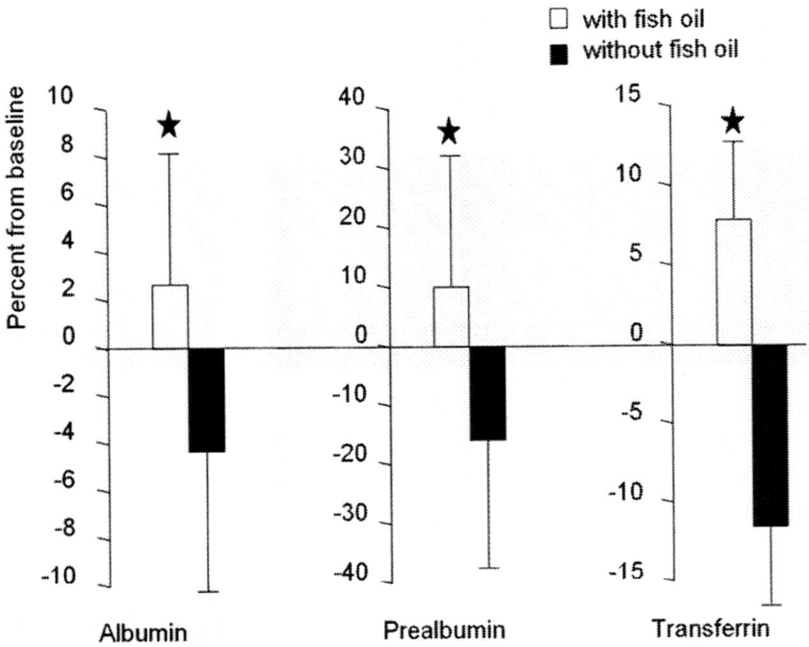

Figure 17. Percentage changes in concentrations of acute phase proteins in weight losing patients with advanced pancreatic cancer given either nutritional supplement enriched with fish oil or full supportive care. Median and interquartile range. The fish oil group received a daily dose of 2.18 g EPA and 0.92 g DHA for 24 d *$p<0.05$ Mann-Whitney U test [9].

Weight loss at baseline of 2.9 kg per month was reversed by EPA. Even a weight gain of 2 kg was achieved after 7 weeks. Moreover, improved activity of natural killer cells, lymphocyte proliferation and increases in CD4/CD8 ratio were observed after fish oil 1.8 g/d during radio-chemotherapy after oesophagectomy [122]. Those effects were underscored by an improvement of markers of the nutritional state, as depicted in figure 17.

3.3. Effects of Intravenous Fish Oil on Pulmonary Integrity and Function

The low prevalence of lung disease among the Greenland Inuit seems to be the result of their diet, which is high in omega-3 FA found in fish oil. Omega-3 FA are rapidly incorporated in cellular membranes of lung tissue and circulating blood cells and replace the omega-6 FA, especially the arachidonic acid (AA). In the case of an inflammatory stimulation omega-3 FA such as eicosapentaenoic acid and docosahexaenoic acid are metabolized via the cyclo- and lipoxygenase pathway into triene prostaglandins and pentaene leukotrienes which have less inflammatory and bronchoconstrictive effects than the corresponding AA-derived lipid mediators. Besides the effects on lipid mediator formation, omega-3 FA modify the function of membrane-linked enzyme systems, signal transduction and receptor functions. Epidemiologic studies have shown potential protective effects against asthma in children, and against emphysema and chronic bronchitis in adults. Acute lung injury was attenuated by omega-3 FA in several clinical studies. In addition, fish oil consumption has been shown to be protective in patients with cystic fibrosis by balancing the abnormal fatty acid metabolism.

3.3.1. Acute Inflammatory Reactions in the Lung

The lung is subject to multiple threats during its physiological function, but in particular during infection and inflammation. The critical pulmonary air-blood interface must deal with a number of problems. Firstly, this interface must be kept tight in both directions allowing diffusible gas exchange, but preventing air bubbles from entering the blood stream and vice versa preventing blood from entering the alveolar space. Further, depending on the degree of body activity, large blood-volume flows are present in the lung vasculature, reflecting the total cardiac output, which is a critical issue in terms of transcapillary filtration and lymph drainage. Except from the lung no other organ has to deal with comparable high blood flow rates through its capillary bed. So, on account of its large alveolar and vascular surfaces a fine balance between vascular tone and mediator generation is required to preserve pulmonary (micro-) structure and function, in particular in critical illness.

Inflammatory reaction is characterized by a stimulation of humoral and cellular mediator systems and a release of a great variety of inflammatory mediators resulting in alterations in microvascular tone and permeability. Lipid mediators, locally activated, are essentially involved in the regulation of these complex actions. The vasodilative properties of AA-derived prostaglandins such as PGE_2 and PGI_2 enhance vascular leakage and consequently contribute to the development of pulmonary edema. Fatty acid peroxides and leukotrienes additionally increase the local permeability and are potent chemoattractants for neutrophil granulocytes. As a result a further accumulation of phagocytes occurs in the pulmonary microcirculation enhancing the local inflammatory reaction and resulting in an impaired gas exchange and lung tissue injury.

3.3.2. Role of Omega-3 FA in Acute Lung Injury

In pulmonary circulation in particular, inflammatory activation of neutrophils induces interactions with the endothelium (selectins and β2-integrins) and release of pro-inflammatory arachidonic acid derivatives resulting in capillary damage, and consequently in increased permeability. These mechanisms are crucial pathogenic factors for the development of acute lung injury and the acute respiratory distress syndrome (ARDS). Omega-3-FA seem to be capable of impeding or inhibiting hyper-inflammatory processes by changing cell-to-cell signal transduction. As described earlier, this is induced by the reduced release of pro-inflammatory arachidonic acid-derivatives and the platelet-activating factor on the one hand,

and the amplification of anti-inflammatory EPA-derivatives on the other hand, which lower the formation of cytokines such as TNFα and IL-1 [99] in monocytes.

The mortality from ARDS still remains high. In recent years numerous experimental and clinical studies were conducted to evaluate new therapeutic strategies in the treatment of acute lung injury/ARDS. Auxiliary approaches such as monoclonal antibodies against pro-inflammatory cytokines and endotoxin have been tested succesfully in experimental studies yet did not show significant effects on patient outcome in clinical studies.

The application of fish oil represents a promising adjuvant strategy because of its anti-inflammatory effects combined with a lower impairment of cellular immune functions such as bacterial clearance and killing as compared to long chain omega-6 FA [73,108]. During inflammation arachidonic acid is released from cellular membranes and metabolized into pro-inflammatory endoperoxides, prostaglandins and leukotrienes.

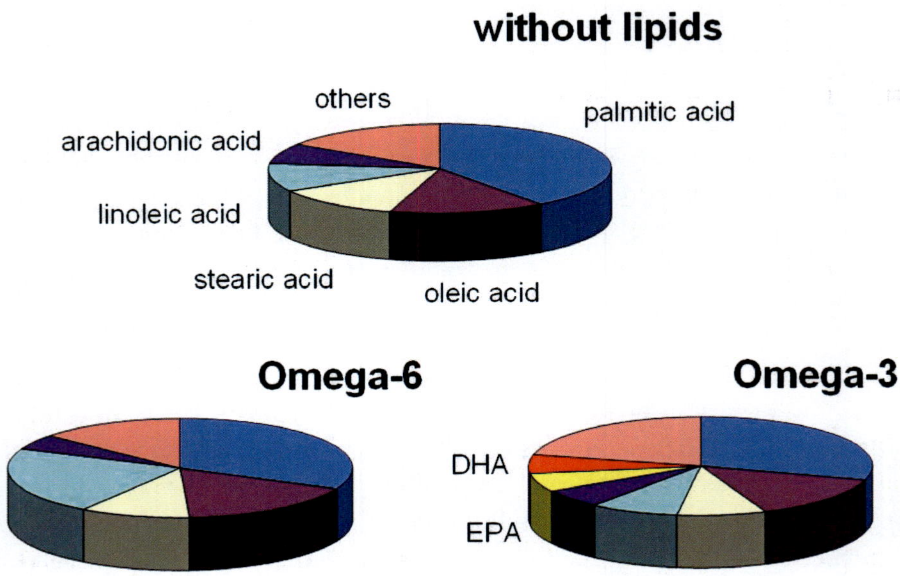

Figure 18. Fatty acid membrane composition in control lungs without lipid perfusion and after 180 min of perfusion with 0.2 g/kg of fish oil or soy bean oil emulsion. Data taken from [20]. (Figures translated and reprinted with permission of Georg Thieme Publishers, Stuttgart, Germany, from Heller AR, et al., AINS 1998)

Improvement of the critically ill was encouraging after replacing arachidonic acid (AA) in cellular membranes with long chain omega-3 FA such as eicosapentaenoic acid and docosahexaenoic acid contained in fish oil [93].

In contrast to the numerous previous studies investigating the effects of a long term (weeks- months) diet containing fish oil [28,29], our interest was focused on the question whether or not omega-3 FA are integrated into the phospholipid pool even after only a short-term intravenous fish oil application, and whether they induce organ protective effects by means of their metabolites after inflammatory stimulation. In a first step we investigated the lipid membrane composition by gas chromatography after a short-term infusion of omega-3

FA [20]. Therefore, we induced a low level inflammatory reaction in isolated and cell-free perfused rabbit lungs by A_{23187} calciumionophore, which triggers AA-metabolism via transmembraneousCa^{2+}- influx as observed after exposure to bacterial toxins. Compared to controls a significant uptake of the omega-3 fatty acids EPA and DHA (figure 18) was observed after only three hours of lung perfusion with a fish oil containing fatty acid emulsion [20]. Moreover, the pulmonary arterial pressure (figure 19) after inflammatory stimulation was considerably blunted during perfusion with omega-3 FA, and was associated with a 50% lower weight increase (figure 20), indicating reduced edema formation [79].

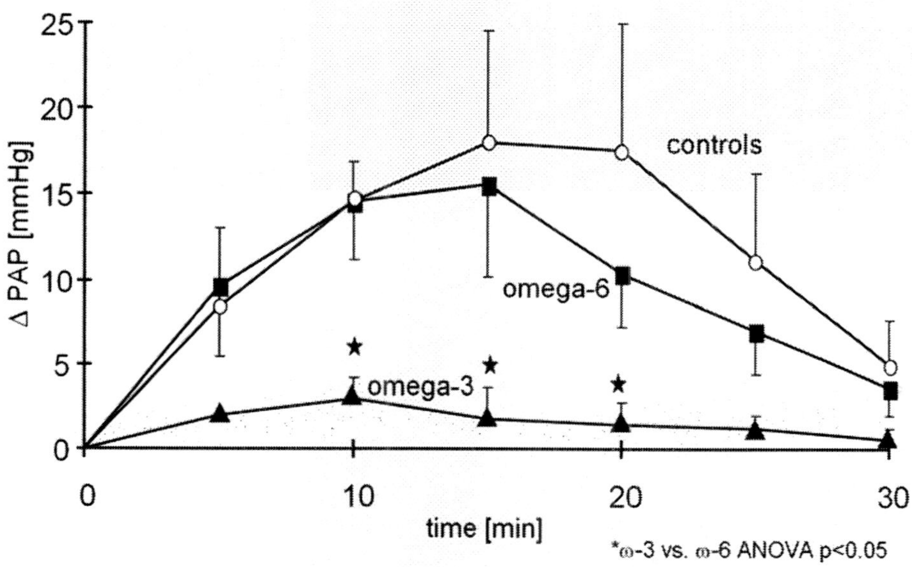

Figure 19. Effects of omega-3 fatty acids on pulmonary artery pressure (PAP) in isolated rabbit lungs under inflammatory stimulation. Data given as pressure increase from baseline [79]. (Figure modified and reprinted with permission of the Publisher www.tandf.co.uk, from Koch T, et al., Clin Intens Care 1993)

The capillary filtration coefficient (Cf_c) describes alterations in vascular permeability and, thus, serves as a measure of vascular leakage. It can be determined when tissue weight gain over time under defined capillary pressures is recorded (figure 21). The estimation of the capillary filtration coefficient is possible using isolated perfused and ventilated rabbit lungs. Closer scrutiny showed different responses to the type of fatty acid applied (figure 22, table 9). As expected, Cf_c values increased after injection of calciumionophore in the control preparations. The lungs perfused with omega-6 FA showed up to 24-fold increases of vascular leakage, whereas fish oil perfusion reduced transcapillary leak from intravascular fluid reflected by Cf_c values which were reduced by up to 50% [81].

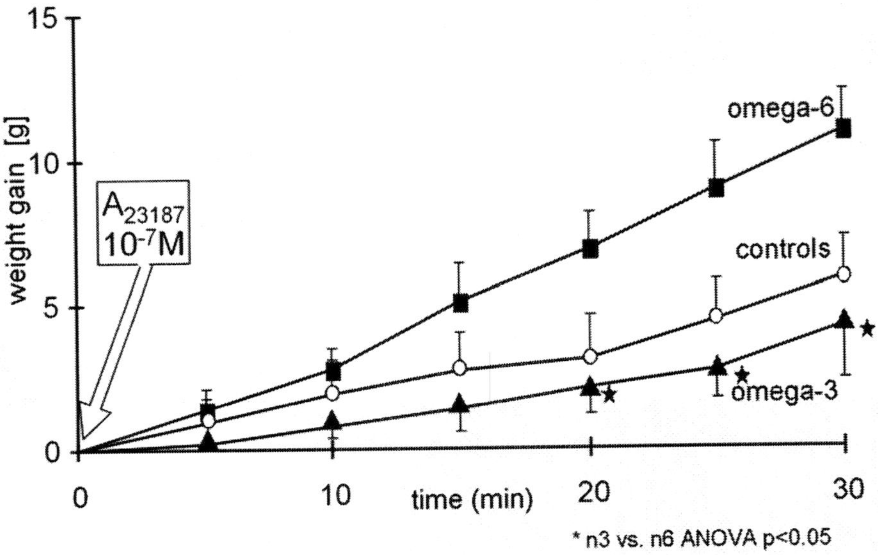

Figure 20. Comparison of lung edema formation in isolated ventilated and perfused rabbit lungs after administration of 0.1g/kg soybean oil (omega-6 FA; n=6) or 0.1g/kg fish oil (omega-3 FA; n=6) emulsion and controls (n=6) [79]. (Modified and reprinted with permission of S. Karger AG Medical and Scientific Publishers, Basel, Switzerland, from Koch T, et al., Infusionsther. Transfusionsmed. 1993)

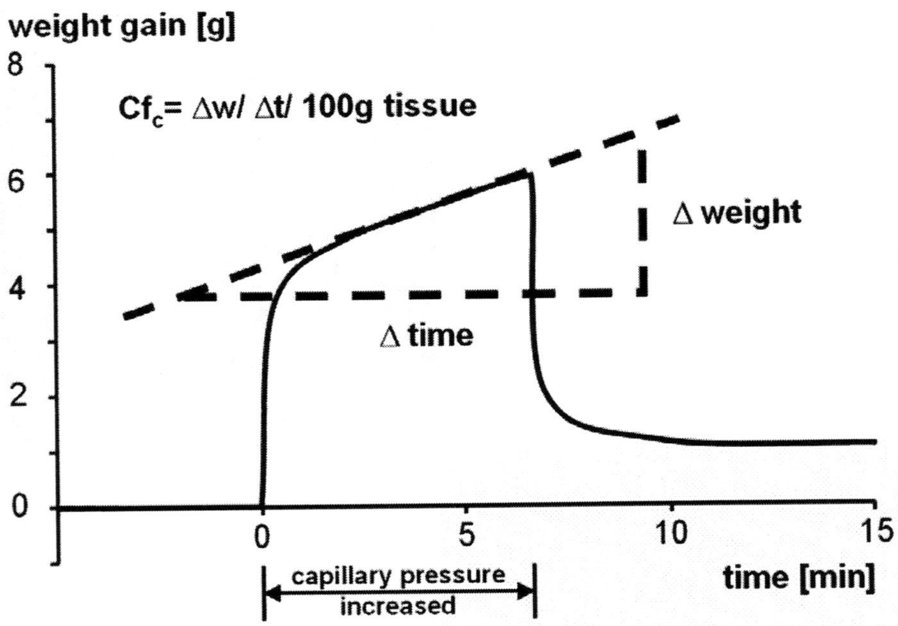

Figure 21. Measurement of capillary filtration coefficients by temporary (7min) increasing capillary afterload (pulmonary venous pressure) under defined preload (perfusion pressure) in isolated lungs. Calculation of the pulmonary weight increase over time enables assumptions regarding transcapillary volume flow and therefore capillary permeability.

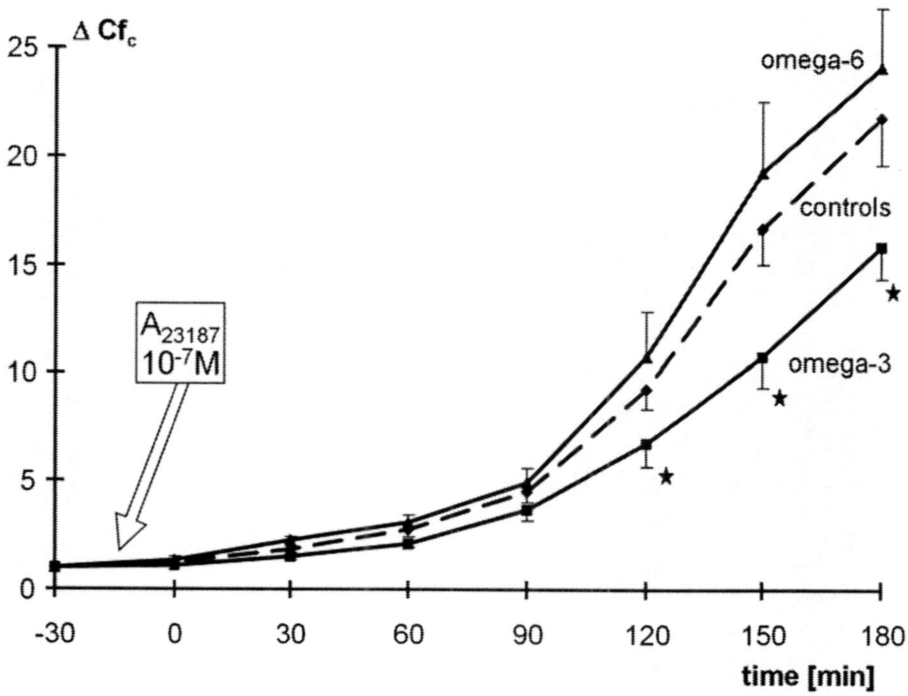

Figure 22. Effects of omega-3 fatty acids on the capillary filtration coefficient (Cf_c) as a measure of capillary permeability in isolated rabbit lungs under inflammatory stimulation. Data given as x-fold increase from baseline [81]. (Figure modified and reprinted with permission of the Publisher www.tandf.co.uk, from Koch T, et al., Clin Intens Care 1995)

Table 9. Impact of differential lipid administration on the development of capillary leakage as reflected by capillary filtration coefficients in isolated rabbit lungs. Timepoint -30 minutes (baseline) was considered 1 and respective timepoints reflect the x-fold increase of capillary filtration coefficients (mean±SD). Inflammatory stimulation with $A_{23187}$was at timepoint -15 [56]

	Time (min)	-30	0	30	60	90	120	150	180
without A_{23}-inflammation	Negative control	1	1.0±0.2	1.1± 0.2	1.5± 0.4	1.8±0.2	2.7± 0.3	3.6±0.4	4.7±0.3
	Omega-6	1	1.0± 0.2	1.4± 0.1	1.9± 0.3	2.6±0.5	4.5±1.0	8.4±2.5	12.2± 3.8
	Omega-3	1	1.0± 0.2	1.2± 0.2	1.7± 0.3	2.7± 0.6	4.4± 1.0	6.1±1.4	7.8± 1.6
A_{23}- inflammation	Positive control	1	1.3±0.2	1.8± 0.2	2.7± 0.3	4.5± 0.7	9.3± 1.0	16.8± 1.3	21.8± 1.8
	Omega-6	1	1.4± 0.1	2.2± 0.2	3.1± 0.3	5.0± 0.6	10.8± 2.1	19.3± 3.3	24.2± 2.8
	Omega-3	1	1.1± 0.1	1.5± 0.1	2.1± 0.2	3.7± 0.5	6.8± 1.1	10.8± 1.4	15.9± 1.6
Neutrophils + A_{23}-inflammation	Omega-6	1	0.67	1.53	3.4	6.33	11.87	24.08	-
	Omega-3	1	1.15	1.62	2.04	3.15	8.70	15.56	-

Similar effects were observed under a plain cell-free perfusion with 1% of lipid emulsion, as well as under lipid perfusion in A_{23187} inflammatory conditions. Most striking were the experimental results indicating the efficacy of omega-3 fatty acids even in the presence of additional neutrophils in the artificial circulation of the isolated lungs, which boosted the vascular damage due to their stimulation by A_{23187}.

These data correlated with the synthesis of EPA- derived cysteinyl-leukotrienes (figure 23), while the AA- derived leukotrienes and thromboxanes were only detectable in small quantities.

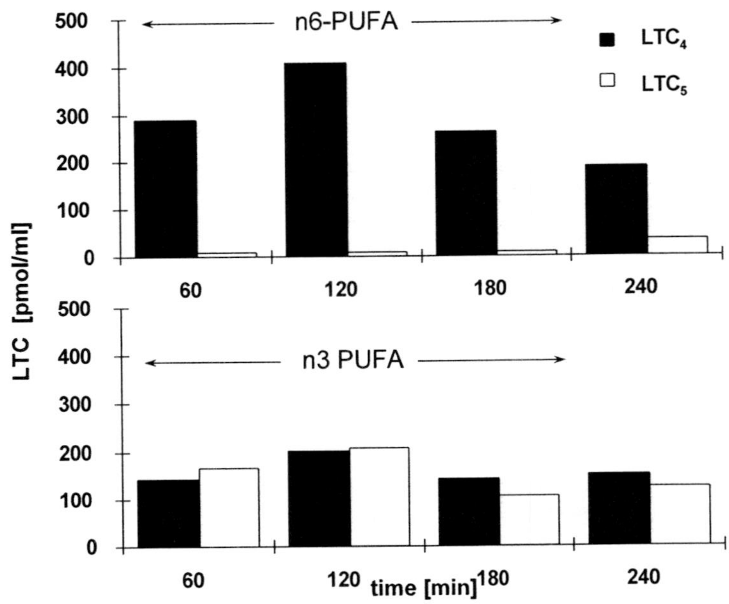

Figure 23. Time course of leukotriene C_4 and C_5 concentrations in the perfusate of isolated ventilated and perfused rabbit lungs after administration of 0.1g/kg soybean oil (omega-6 FA; n=6) or 0.1g/kg fish oil (omega-3 FA; n=6) emulsion [56,81]. (Figure modified and reprinted with permission of the Publisher www.tandf.co.uk, from Koch T, et al., Clin Intens Care 1995)

Compared to controls, treatment with omega-3 FA did not influence release of vasodilatory prostacyclin. These results suggest a relevant uptake of EPA into lung tissue after 3 hours of perfusion and metabolization of EPA due to inflammatory activation.

The clinical impact of these findings [20,56,78,79] was very well demonstrated in 146 patients with ARDS by Gadek and the „Enteral Nutrition in ARDS Study Group" in 1999 [38]. Due to the improvement of the pulmonary gas exchange lower inspiratory oxygen concentrations and inferior levels of positive endexspiratory pressure were sufficient to assure adequate oxygen delivery (DO_2) compared to controls. Weaning times from the respirator and ICU dismissal occurred in significantly shorter time after fish oil application. Re- evaluation of the patients serum from this study revealed reduced humoral host response in terms of IL-6, IL-8, TNFα, and LTB_4 and gave the biochemical and pathophysiological rationale for the clinically observed improvement of the pulmonary condition [104] as postulated by our group from experimental studies [20,56,78,79].

In view of clinical consequences, these findings point toward prophylactic and therapeutic effects in inflammatory diseases and acute lung injury [3], which seem to be attainable by a simple rearrangement of nutritional components. Finally, recent recommendations by the Canadian Society for Nutrition recognize the evidence based therapeutic value of omega-3 FA in acute respiratory distress [62].

3.4. Effects of Fish Oil on Liver Function

Following major abdominal non-liver surgery increases in ALAT were observed and correlated with ultrastructural damage of the liver [90]. In the postoperative phase after major abdominal surgery, an intact liver function is crucial not only for energy balance (glucose and lactate metabolism) but also for providing several humoral factors, which a) induce, b) support, and c) ultimately terminate regenerative mechanisms. This acute phase response (APR) of the liver sets on immediately after the (surgical) trauma and primarily, up-regulates coagulation factors and proteinase inhibitors for the healing process, and complement components and opsonins (C-reactive protein) for early bactericidal activity at the site of trauma [14]. If properly regulated, APR is self-terminating upon completion of the reparatory activity of the organism [17]. Under certain circumstances such as the systemic inflammatory response syndrome (SIRS) or sepsis APR may get out of control and may consequently damage host tissue by overwhelming activation [45,58,132].

Poeze and colleagues demonstrated that increased transaminases and bilirubin precede the onset of organ dysfunction after elective high-risk surgery [106] and hyperbilirubinaemia was associated with a two-fold duration of ICU-stay [67] and an increased incidence of complications after esophageal resection [126]. Moreover, inadequate hyperactivation of the APR in patients with unresectable pancreatic cancer was associated with reduced survival [35].

After administering omega-3 FA Pscheidl found improved splanchnic perfusion and increased lactate clearance in the liver [109]. In addition, this group provided evidence for enhanced hepatic immune competence in terms of bactericidal capacity after fish oil intakes during endotoxemia [108]. Based on these data and on the notion that rapid effects of omega-3 FA can be achieved within a few days, we hypothesized, that administering fish oil emulsion might improve the liver function in patients undergoing surgical procedures for treatment of upper gastrointestinal cancer [84]. Early convalescence of liver function boosts host defense, the coagulation system, and protein synthesis required for wound healing. Patient recovery, in particular in those patients at risk for the development of a systemic inflammatory response in the postoperative phase should therefore accelerate. Such individuals were identified by determining the ratio of interleukin (IL)-6/ IL-10 on postoperative day one. This ratio reported by Tanigushi reflects the pro- and anti-inflammatory balance and showed a close correlation with the incidence of septic complications in the subsequent clinical phase [121].

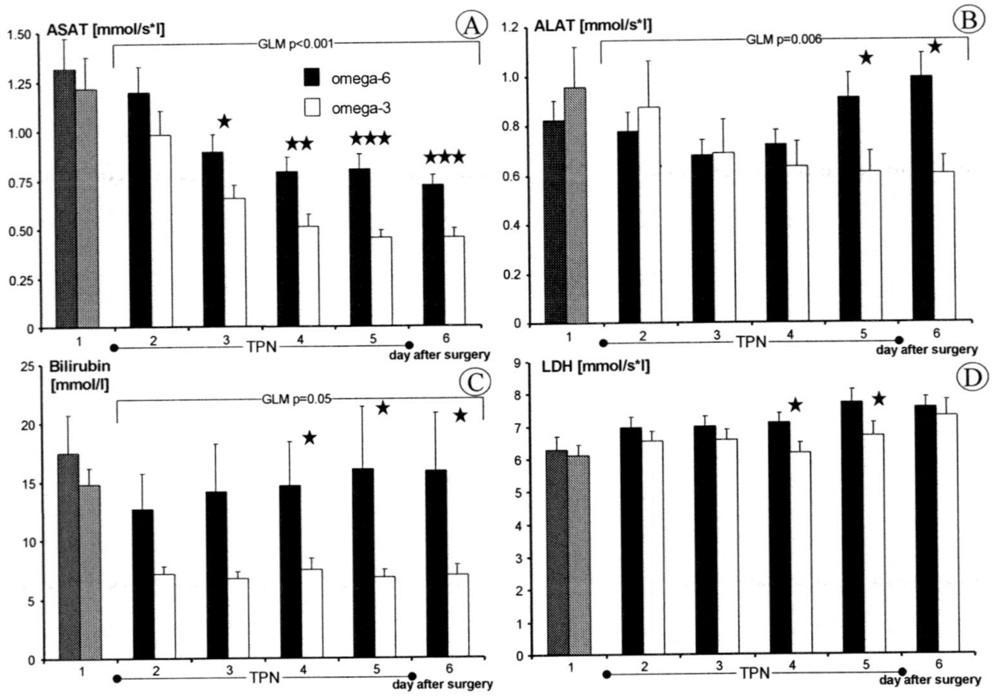

Figure 24. A) Aspartataminotransferase (ASAT), B) Alaninaminotransferase (ALAT) C) Bilirubin D) Lactatedehydrogenase (LDH) (means ±SEM) after major abdominal cancer surgery followed by total parenteral nutrition (TPN) supplemented with soybean oil (omega-6, black columns) or with fish oil (omega-3, white columns) emulsions. *Post hoc* Bonferroni adjusted daily comparison: * $p<0.05$; ** $p<0.01$; *** $p<0.001$; hatched columns baseline before TPN [60]. (Reprinted with permission, International Journal of Cancer © copyright (2004) Wiley-Liss Inc., from Heller AR, et al.)

Compared to a single parenteral supplementation with SO, an additional FO application resulted in a significant decrease of the liver enzymes ASAT and ALAT as well as of bilirubin over the whole observation period. Moreover, lactatdehydrogenase was reduced on days four and five in the omega-3 group and, thus, exhibited liver protective effects.

The liver enzymes ASAT and ALAT as well as their ratio significantly increased after surgery. Hence, serum levels of ASAT may be confounded by surgery-associated tissue injury and may, therefore, not exclusively reflect the hepatic condition. Considering type and duration of the surgical procedure, the occurrence of tissue trauma was distributed homogeneously in both groups.

Similar effects were reported in septic mice by Hwang and co-workers, who found reduced liver enzymes and mortality after FO administration, which was attributed to down-regulation of hepatocellular apoptosis [69]. Regarding splanchnic vasculature Pscheidl demonstrated improved perfusion and fewer translocation of viable bacteria from the gut into mesenteric lymph nodes and the liver after omega-3 fatty acids [116]. This mechanism could have contributed to the beneficial effects on pancreas and liver after TPN supplemented with FO.

One of the immuno-stimulant FO-effects was the amplification of the "positive hepatic acute phase response" [115], as measured by CRP and fibrinogen. This immune-augmentation could in part be attributed to the improved liver-function which was reflected by lower transaminases bilirubin and lactatdehydrogenase. The strengthened hepatic production of proteins of humoral host defense or of coagulation factors [105] correlates with higher serum-levels of opsonizing CRP or fibrinogen. Conversely, a weakened acute-phase reaction after burn injury was associated with elevated mortality rates [18]. However, the issue of the acute phase response seems to be cutting both ways. The APR is a condition *sine qua non* for initiating repair mechanisms in states of a properly regulated inflammatory response, as observed in the early recovery from burn injury [20], or in the current postoperative patients. If on the other hand an inadequately prolonged or overwhelming APR is present as in advanced sepsis [20,34] or in patients with tumor cachexia [43] the APR turns from friend to foe. The APR then itself becomes a part of the pathomechanism and may induce an unfavorable outcome.

In addition, a weight loss of 1.1 kg was found after SO which was completely stopped in the FO+SO- group, despite a 0.5 l lower cumulative ICU fluid balance after FO+SO. Similar improvements of the nutritional state in cachectic cancer patients receiving omega-3 FA were recently reported by Barber and colleagues [29]. Weight loss at baseline of 2.9 kg per month was reversed by omega-3 FA. Even weight gain at both 3 (median 1 kg) and 7 weeks (median 2 kg) was achieved.

3.4.1. Effects of Omega-3 Fatty Acids on Metabolism

Martina Wendel and Axel Heller

During the acute phase response, marked metabolic alterations are observed. Acute conditions such as surgical trauma, inflammation, and sepsis induce major changes in the concentration, composition, and metabolism of plasma lipoproteins as well as increases in serum glucose levels due to insulin resistance. Changes in lipid metabolism are reflected by increased serum triglyceride (TG) levels and decreases in total cholesterol as well as high- and low-density lipoproteins, HDL and LDL. Concomitantly with enhanced TG levels, VLDL levels in plasma rise. In this context, elevated TG levels and free fatty acids delivered to peripheral tissues such as skeletal muscle are known to impair insulin signaling and also contribute to the development of insulin resistance.

Large epidemiologic studies demonstrated that omega-3 FA like eicosapentaeonic acid (EPA) and docosahexaeonic acid (DHA) improve the profile of serum lipids [29]. They decreased TG levels and increased HDL cholesterol while total cholesterol and LDL levels remained constant or decreased slightly. These changes were accompanied by a reduced cardiovascular risk. Omega-3 FA were also reported to ameliorate insulin resistance, however, these results are controversial at present. The changes in lipid metabolism, nonetheless, seem to be of clinical relevance. Elevated TG levels correlated linearly with mortality in surgical ICU patients and reductions in both HDL lipoprotein and total cholesterol were associated with poor clinical outcome, infectious complications, and increased concentrations of proinflammatory cytokines in critically ill patients. Lipoproteins are thought to be important regulators of the host immune response due to their lipopolysaccharide (LPS)-neutralizing capacities. Lipoproteins were essential for the release of bound LPS from cell membranes and HDL was the main lipoprotein involved, while binding of LPS occurred mainly by LDL and VLDL in serum and by VLDL in the lymph of septic individuals. In addition, lipoproteins exert antiinflammatory actions by modulation of adhesion molecule expression, endothelial nitric oxide production and antioxidant properties.

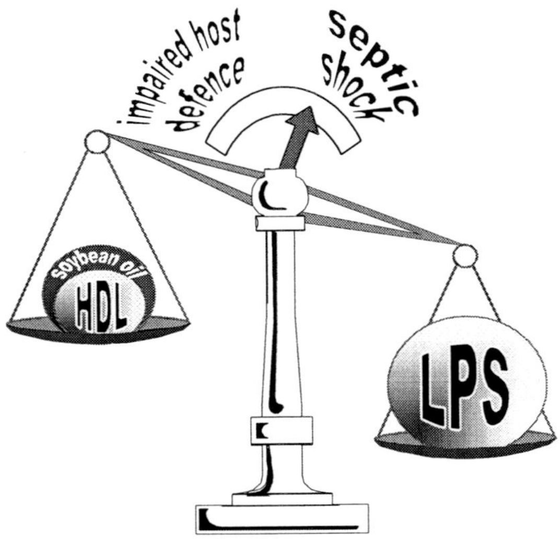

Figure 25. Double edged sword: While endotoxin (LPS) promotes septic shock, up to now it is unclear if LPS neutralizing therapeutic approaches with HDL or with soy bean oil based lipid emulsions may impair host defence.

Substitution of lipoproteins by infusion of reconstituted HDL (rHDL) has been proposed as therapeutic option. In animal models of endotoxemia, application of rHDL decreased mortality. In humans, infusion of rHDL blunted endotoxin-induced procoagulant activation without adverse side effects. However, safety of rHDL application is a concern as infusion of higher doses of rHDL has been demonstrated to promote growth of candida albicans ex vivo although the clinical significance of this finding is currently unknown.

One ongoing worldwide multicenter trial recruiting more than 1,800 patients with gram-negative sepsis tries to establish the therapeutic efficacy of intravenous lipid administration on LPS neutralisation. The proposed mechanism of action is to expand the phospholipid surface on plasma lipiproteins e.g. HDL and thereby facilitating LPS neutralisation. Similar to rHDL, soy bean oil emulsions (omega-6 FA) have, likewise, been claimed to be associated with infectious complications [63]. Thus, the concept of administration of soybean oil as well as of rHDL seems to be double edged and has to be considered cautiously, in particular in patients with suspected infection. In this regard, lipid emulsions with a reduced content of omega-6 FA in favour of medium chain TG, or olive oil, or fish oil rich in omega-3 FA may be the better choice. Recently Lekka and coworkers reported that total parenteral nutrition with medium-chain and long-chain triglycerides aggravated lung inflammation and deteriorated gas exchange in patients with ARDS. However, the adverse effects observed in their study might at least in part be due to to the rapid infusion rate used. From animal experimental data, inclusion of omega-3 FA may be useful in attenuating lipid induced pulmonary inflammation in acute lung injury [20,78,79]

Although the LPS-neutralizing effects of lipoproteins and apolipoprotein mimetic peptides are well characterized, the significance of these mechanisms in the context of bacterial infections is not as clear. Flegel and coworkers demonstrated that the LPS-neutralizing capacity of lipoproteins does not correlate with the inhibition of cytokine release induced by whole gram-negative bacteria in vitro. So, the efficacy of therapeutic approaches aiming at neutralizing LPS by the use of lipoproteins and apolipoprotein mimetic peptides has to be evaluated carefully in the clinical setting in patients with bacterial infections.

In epidemiologic studies, omega-3 FA were reported to increase plasma levels of HDL cholesterol. As HDL cholesterol is negatively regulated during the APR and due to its role in the release of bound LPS from cell membranes, amelioration of the APR-induced decline in plasma HDL-levels by dietay supplementation of omega-3 FA would be favourable.

We observed reductions in both HDL- and LDL-cholesterol which were maximal at the second postoperative day. HDL-cholesterol did not significantly change during the course of TPN and did not differ between the two treatment groups [60]. So, omega-3 FA obviously are not capable of influencing the APR-induced downregulation of HDL cholesterol. LDL-cholesterol increased in both treatment groups and was significantly higher in the omega-3 group compared to the omega-6 group. In the case of VLDL, we observed elevations in both groups (figure 26). Elevation of hepatic TG synthesis and VLDL secretion are characteristic for the APR and are also promoted by exogenous administration of highly unsaturated fatty acids. In addition, apoE is negatively regulated during the APR. Reduced expression of apoE leads to decreased apoE content of VLDL and diminished VLDL clearance ultimately resulting in elevated VLDL levels. So, increases in VLDL might in part be caused by decreased clearance of VLDL.

Concerning the regulation of hepatic TG and VLDL secretion, omega-3 FA take an exceptional position among polyunsaturated fatty acids as studies both in healthy human subjects and in in vitro cell culture experiments demonstrated an inhibitory effect of omega-3 FA on VLDL secretion. At the cellular level, most studies showed that omega-3 FA inhibited hepatocellular apoB and VLDL secretion while the extent varied with the cell type and species studied. In contrast we observed increased VLDL levels in patients receiving omega-3 FA, while TG levels did not differ significantly between the two groups. This may allow the conclusion the inhibitory effect of omega-3 FA on hepatic VLDL secretion is not present during the early postoperative course after major abdominal surgery. Rather, we observed an immediate rise in VLDL levels in the omega-3 FA group whereas the increase in VLDL levels seems to be delayed in the omega-6 FA group. After one week of TPN the difference in VLDL levels between omega-3 and omega-6 FA treatment disappeared and glycerol levels were significantly lower in the omega-3 versus the omega-6 FA group.

Compared with day 5 of TPN, VLDL levels decreased in the omega-3 FA group while they increased in the omega-6 FA group. From these observations, one might speculate that the VLDL-lowering effect of omega-3 FA is offset by acute regulatory changes during the APR and that the early rise in VLDL levels induced by TPN including omega-3 FA may reflect improvements in liver function in these patients, which have been reported previously [60]. In this context, changes in the hepatocellular redox state during the acute phase response might contribute to the observed increase in VLDL by omega-3 FA. Because VLDL similar to HDL may, likewise, serve as a LPS scavenger fish oil supplementation should be considered for that purpose in severe illness, rather than plain soybean oil which prolongs bacterial elimination compared to fish oil.

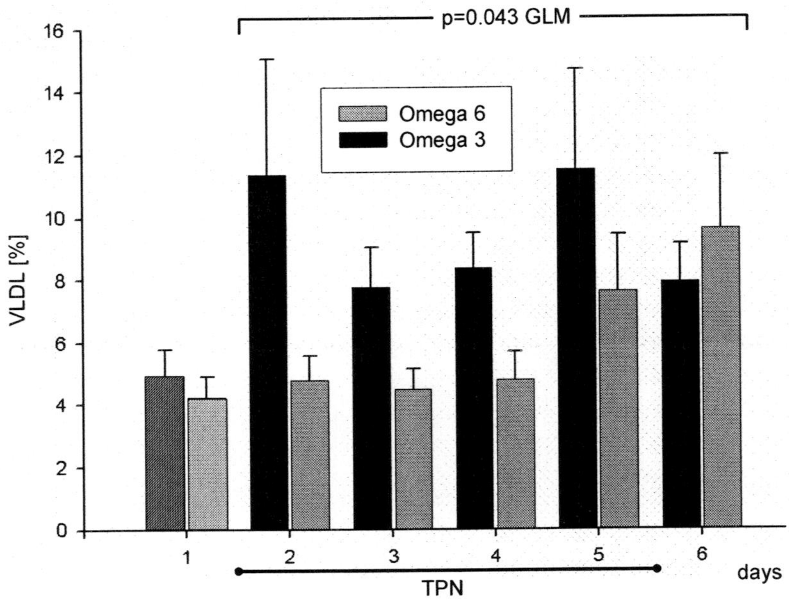

Figure 26. Very low density lipoprotein (VLDL) in % of lipoproteins after major abdominal cancer surgery followed by total parenteral nutrition (TPN) supplemented with soybean oil (omega-6, black columns) or with fish oil (omega-3, grey columns) emulsions; hatched columns baseline before TPN.

VLDL are assembled in two steps. The first involves transfer of lipid by the microsomal transfer protein (MTP) to apoB during translation. In the second step apoB-containing precursor particles are fused with triglyceride droplets to form mature VLDL. In addition, cholesteryl-esters are transferred to VLDL particles via ACAT2. Secretion of VLDL is controlled primarily at the level of presecretory degradation by two distinct mechanisms: the first is called ER-associated degradation (ERAD) and uptake which commits newly synthesized apoB 100 to degradation and is effective mainly under conditions when lipid supply is limited. She second is so-called post-ER presecretory proteolysis (PERPP) which targets lipid-rich apoB-lipoproteins and decreases their secretion. Polyunsaturated fatty acids have been demonstrated to increase PERPP by a mechanism involving fatty acid-dependent lipid peroxidation, thereby decreasing apoB100 and VLDL secretion. As this pathway is targeted by both omega-3 and omega-6 FA, differences between the two lipid preparations probably not occur at that level but might be causative for the increases in VLDL seen in both groups by TPN. In contrast, specific effects of omega-3 versus omega-6 FA were reported at the level of gene transcription and these were dependent on the hepatocellular redox state. While under normal redox conditions, omega-3 FA did not affect apoB, MTP, or DGAT expression, they increased MTP expression under pro-oxidant and stimulated both MTP and apoB expression under pro-reducing conditions. These changes could ultimately lead to the observed increases in hepatic VLDL secretion in response to omega-3 FA. This hypothesis is supported by the findings of Antebi and coworkers who reported improved plasma antioxidant capacity by parenteral nutrition including omega-3 FA.

The fact that the increase in VLDL secretion by omega-3 FA was not accompanied by a rise in plasma TG levels might be caused by changes in the relative VLDL content of TGs and apoB 100. In primary hepatocytes, a PPARα agonist decreased synthesis and secretion of TGs in the face of increased synthesis of apoB 100 and lead to the formation of smaller VLDL particles which contained fewer TGs and more apoB 100. As omega-3 FA are known ligands of PPARs, this might explain the differential effects of omega-3 FA on VLDL and TG levels in our study.

Omega-3 FA exert diverse effects on a large number of cell types thereby modulating immune function, proinflammatory signaling, as well as glucose and lipid metabolism. Inclusion of omega-3 FA into both enteral as well as parenteral nutrition of critically ill patients lead to improved outcome and also reduced costs [12,38,41,107]. While improvements in cellular immunity and organ function as well as attenuation of hyperinflammatory states and infectious complications by omega-3 FA in critically ill patients have been reported previously, the impact of short-term parenteral nutrition including omega-3 FA on glucose and lipid homeostasis during the postoperative period has not been characterized. Studies in insulin-resistant and obese individuals demonstrated that long-term oral intake of omega-3 FA ameliorated elevated TG levels and had an inhibitoy effect on hepatic VLDL apoB secretion. In rats, increased beta-oxidation of fatty acids primarily in the liver but also in skeletal muscle tissue were shown to contribute to the hypotriglyceridemic effect of dietary omega-3 FA and this was accompanied by enhanced insulin sensitivity. In addition, omega-3 FA were shown to enhance peripheral glucose deposition due to increased glucose uptake by skeletal muscle. In this regard, elevated plasma TG levels correlated with mortality in post-cardiac surgery patients. Elevated plasma TG levels also contribute to peripheral insulin resistance by impairing insulin-receptor signaling ultimately leading to decreased glucose uptake by skeletal muscle cells and serum hyperglycemia. So, lowering of plasma TG by omega-3 FA might be favourable during the postoperative course and could promote a more rapid recovery of metabolic homeostasis. However, studies in insulin-resistant human individuals who received omega-3 FA for a prolonged period are controversial: while in most studies glucose homeostasis was not affected by a diet including omega-3 FA, both improvements and deterioration of glycemic control were reported by others.

One further aspect of the acute phase response is insulin resistance of liver and skeletal muscles resulting in increased hepatic gluconeogenesis, glycogenolysis and reduced peripheral cellular glucose uptake. Elevated TG levels are attributed to enhance peripheral insulin resistance due to interference with insulin-receptor signaling leading to reduced expression of glucose transporter 4 at the cell surface and reduced uptake of glucose by skeletal muscle cells. Long-term studies in humans suggested that omega-3 FA improve glycemic control by two independent mechanisms. First, they were shown to lower serum TG levels and second, they enhanced cellular glucose deposition. However, studies in insulin-resistant patients also reported adverse effects of omega-3 FA on glycemic control.

In postoperative patients, we observed significantly higher serum glucose levels when a TPN including omega-3 FA was applied compared with TPN containing omega-6 FA alone [60]. As daily insulin doses did not differ significantly between the two groups we assume that omega-3 FA exerted a diabetogenic effect and worsened the APR-induced insulin resistance. The increases in serum glucose levels occurred in light of elevated VLDL levles in the omega-3 FA group. However, plasma TG levels did not differ between groups. So, this factor does not seem to contribute to the observed differences between the two lipid preparations. Omega-3 FA have repeatedly been shown to enhance peripheral glucose uptake. However, they also were reported to impair suppression of hepatic endogenous glucose production. In an experimental study in rats, Holness and coworkers demonstrated that feeding a high fat diet which included omega-3 FA improved peripheral glucose disposal compared to a diet with omega-6 FA. But they also showed that inclusion of omega-3 FA impaired insulin-induced suppression of hepatic endogenous glucose production reflecting enhanced hepatic insulin resistance. In addition, inclusion of omega-3 FA lowered the fat-induced basal insulin-secretion of isolated pancreatic islets and augmented the clearance rate of exogenously infused insulin. All together, these mechanisms might account for the significantly elevated serum glucose levels observed in our patients treated with TPN including omega-3 FA. However, the underlying mechanisms and intracellular pathways involved are currently poorly understood.

3.5. Impact of Omega-3 Fatty Acids on Perioperative Hemostasis

Compared to European controls, decreased levels of myocardial infarction in Greenland Inuit, as observed in early epidemiological studies [28,29,30], were attributed to an increase in bleeding time and changes of platelet aggregation after the dietary intake of omega-3 FA contained in fish oil. More recent publications, however, report no [119] or clinically irrelevant [111] changes in platelet aggregation.

Because of beneficial effects on the outcome of severely ill patients [12,38] and the controversial issue of hemostasis during omega-3 FA administration [76] we investigated whether supplementation with FO affects platelet function and plasma haemostatic standard factors in patients after major elective gastrointestinal surgery. The ensuing differential examinations of FO- effects on the intrinsic and extrinsic activation of the coagulation system were done by measuring the activated coagulation factors VII and XII.

Bleeding complications were comparably low in both groups, regardless of the type of fatty acid infused. Preoperatively measured hemoglobin concentrations declined during surgery. Minimum values were reached at day three, but no untoward effects of fish oil were observed. Postoperatively transfused amounts of packed red blood cells showed no difference between soy bean oil and fish oil groups. The administration of fresh frozen plasma (FFP), however, was more frequent in the omega-6 group. Underlying causes for this observation in favor of FO cannot be found in the laboratory measurements, but rather in the physician's decisions being based upon the individual clinical aspect.

Classical hemostasis parameters such as PT, aPTT, platelet counts and AT III were measured prior to surgery and before starting the lipid infusion (table 10). These values were expectedly altered after a major abdominal surgical procedure, indicating a moderate activation of coagulation. The surgical trauma reduced PT and increased aPTT. Under the differential application of omega-3 and omega-6 FA there were no significant differences between groups over time and baseline values were regained between day three and four after surgery. During this time daily anti- thrombotic heparin administration was adjusted to achieve aPTT between 35 and 40s. The required dosages of heparin were comparable in both groups and were increased from day one to day six reflecting the improvement of the coagulation system. Postoperative levels of fibrinogen and AT III revealed no significant between-group differences.

Table 10. Coagulation parameters (mean±SD) before surgery, first day after surgery, and after five days of pareneral nutrition with soybean oil emulsion or fish oil emulsion
n.m not measured. Heparin dosages were adjusted to a PTT of 35-40s. [1]Volumes within the complete postoperative period until day 6

	before surgery	day 1 after surgery		day 6 after surgery	
		Omega-6	Omega-3	Omega-6	Omega-3
prothrombin time [%]	103±13	70±14	72±8	98±14	97±12
PTT [s]	33±4	47±10	44±7	36±12	33±5
Heparin [I.U./d]	15,000	10,300±3,600	10,100±4,200	14,600±2,700	13,500±3,800
Fibrinogen [g/l]	n.m.	3,1±0,7	3,1±0,7	5,5±1,3	6,2±1,7
Antithrombin III [%]	n.m.	68±16	66±11	86±14	85±18
Platelets [GPt l^{-1}]	227±101	193±73	177±90	287±97	295±106
Hemoglobin [mmol/l]	7.7±1.4	6.8±0.9	6.4±1.1	6.6±0.7	6.3±0.9
Hematocrit	0.37±0.07	0.33±0.04	0.31±0.05	0.32±0.03	0.30±0.04
Packed red cells [ml]	-	317±787[1]	325±405[1]	-	-
Fresh froz. plasm.[ml]	-	156±311[1]	42±167[1]	-	-

While omega-3 FA modulate the cytokine expression [26,32,99], PUFA-dependent effects on tissue factor (TF) expression and the extrinsic coagulation pathway were further differentiated by quantifying the activated factor VII. When TF is presented to plasma components during vascular injury, extrinsic coagulation is activated. Factor VIIa and its cofactor TF assemble on a negatively charged membrane surface in a Ca^{2+}-dependent manner to form an enzyme compound which proteolytically converts factor X into Xa [6]. As depicted in figure 27a surgical trauma accelerates factor VIIa-induced clotting, reflecting an elevated level of the activated factor VII and a postoperative (day 1) hypercoagulatory extrinsic state, but preoperative values were regained on day 3. Fish oil administration at the concentration used in this study, however, did not interfere with TF/VIIa activation.

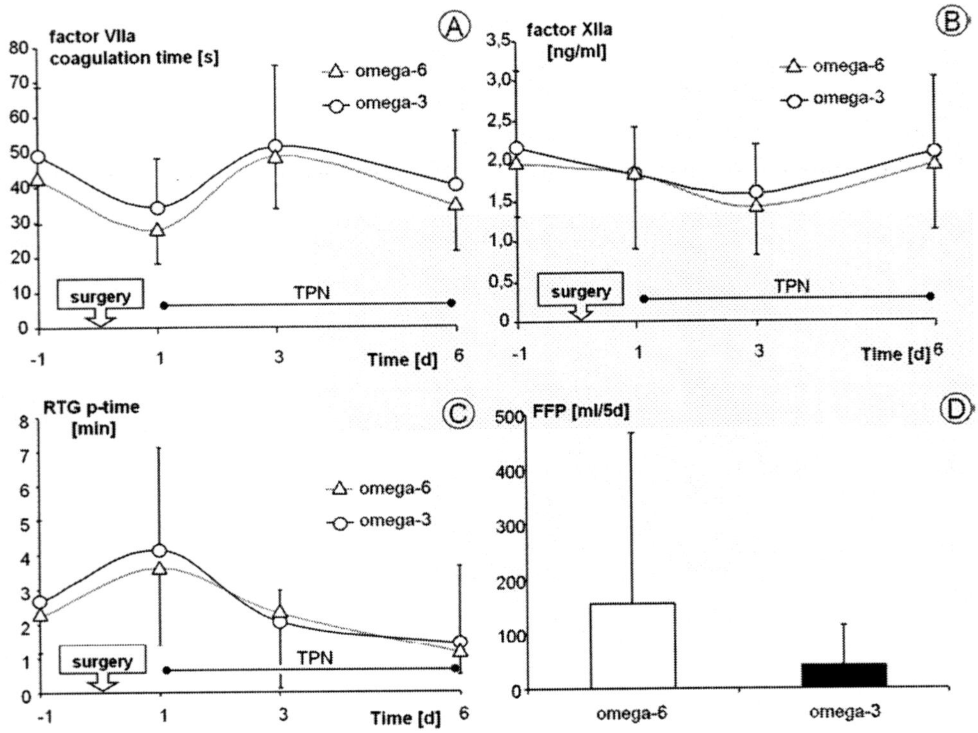

Figure 27. (A) Factor VIIa induced clotting time, (B) Factor XIIa, (C) downward slope period (min) in resonance thrombography (RTG) = platelet induced clot retraction (p)- time (D) use of fresh frozen plasma for substitution of coagulation factors (mean±SD) in 44 patients after major abdominal surgery followed by total parenteral nutrition (TPN) for 5 days supplemented with soybean oil or with fish oil.

The influence of fatty acid administration on intrinsic coagulation was investigated by measuring the activated factor XII (figure 27b), which is a component of the contact system of blood coagulation which also includes prekallikrein, HMW kininogen and factor XI. Because the main physiological activators of factor XII include fatty acids and the surface of certain types of lipoprotein particles [97], the analysis of factor XIIa during differential PUFA administration was of particular interest. In contrast to its effect on extrinsic factor VIIa, surgical trauma was of minor influence for intrinsic factor XIIa levels. Moreover, differential PUFA administration had no impact on XIIa formation.

Despite a drop of platelet counts during surgery no differences were observed between the two study groups; both regained baseline values on postoperative day three. Further, platelet function which was delayed postoperatively, as analyzed by resonance thrombography (RTG) was not affected by FO (figure 27c). During RTG coagulation is mechanically activated in whole blood according to physiological conditions of blood current and intravascular shear stress. In measuring coagulation on the basis of the resonance effect induced by the elastic fibrin structure the RTG principle [52] differes from thrombelastographs [96]. Information about velocity and quality of clot formation is drawn from a specific graph. Distinct segments of the RTG plot represent fibrin formation (f-time = duration of upward slope) or platelet function (p-time = duration of downward slope). RTG p-time reflects the functionality of platelet-derived coagulation, regardless of the underlying cause of platelet malfunction (low platelets, uraemia, fibrinogen cleavage products). Reduced levels of platelet activating factor (PAF) due to omega-3 FA, as reported by Sperling [118] may, thus, be of minor impact in the current clinical setting. Postoperative delay in RTG p-time may reflect dilution effects due to intravenous fluids.

Summarizing our results, global parameters for the assessing the quality of coagulation and haemostasis, such as hemoglobin levels or the demand for packed red blood cells were in accordance with both, basic and advanced coagulation parameters were independent of differential PUFA administration. Fish oil administered up to 0.2 g/kg/d, was shown to be safe in terms of intrinsic and extrinsic coagulation and did not influence platelet aggregation.

3.6. Enteral Nutrition in Patients with Systemic Inflammatory Reaction (SIRS)

Sepsis is a multi-factor condition describing the co-occurrence of infection and a systemic inflammatory reaction (SIRS). Criteria for SIRS are fever or hypothermia, leukocytosis or leukopenia, tachycardia and tachypnea. If one or more vital organs (i.e. heart, kidney, lung, liver) fail in addition to sepsis the patient's condition is defined as a severe sepsis. Septic shock is defined as sepsis complicated by low blood pressure and which is refractory to fluid therapy [86,87].

Although no single agent or treatment strategy for sepsis is known up to date a decrease in mortality among postoperative and posttraumatic sepsis patients could be observed over the past years [37]. This can be attributed to modern intensive care treatment with early enteral nutrition, avoidance of nosocomial infections as well as stress ulcers and to thromboembolism prophylaxis [87].

Nutritional therapy therefore has become a focus of intensive care physicians in the treatment of sepsis in addition to basic therapy. The main goal of modern nutrition therapy is to offer patients nutrition specially adapted to metabolic demands (substrate guided, overflow limited). Van den Berge et al. showed that a hyperalimentation in terms of hyperglycemia is deleterious and normoglycemia (glucose <6.1 mmol/l, <110 mg/dl) should be maintained. In a study including 1548 ventilated patients normoglycemia as opposed to a liberal blood glucose regime (glucose <11 mmol/l, <200 mg/dl) led to a significant reduction in ventilator days, intensive care therapy stay and mortality.

The metabolism of patients in physiological conditions is quite different from metabolic processes in states of starvation and (postagression) stress response. In starvation substrate use is not disturbed and a catabolic state can therefore easily be reversed by an adequate substrate supply. The goal of malnutrition therapy is to restore body cell mass. Stress induces a mediator- and hormone- induced disturbance of substrate utilization and an increase in metabolic rate (hypermetabolism). In this case exogenous substrate supply is not or just barely able to influence the mobilization of energy and substrate reserves. Stress metabolism is divided into two main phases: The ebb phase (early phase) and the flow phase.

The ebb phase (immediately after injury, 0-36 h) is a direct response to a stimulus such as trauma and is characterized by high plasma catecholamine, cortisol and glucagon levels. Catecholamines lead to an improved organ perfusion, thereby also increasing the energy supply. At the same time cortisol release leads to an increase in sodium and water retention. The metabolism of energy reserves is switched to gluconeogenesis: body protein is broken down for a synthesis of acute phase proteins and glucose. The stabilization of disturbed vital functions is the main focus of intensive care therapy in this phase. Additional nutritional therapy at this point leads to metabolic stress [103].

12-36 hours after injury the ebb phase is followed by the flow phase, mainly dominated by the sympathetic nervous system. Patients in this phase often have high blood glucose levels as a sign of disturbed carbohydrate utilization. The flow phase results in a redistribution of glucose in favor of the insulin-independent uptake in brain tissue. Increased plasma cortisol levels inhibiting pyruvate- dehydrogenase and increased availability of free fatty acids seem to be the basis for peripheral insulin resistance. Metabolic changes are induced by the increased release of free radicals, pro-inflammatory eicosanoids, interleukins and TNF. IL 1 for instance increases cellular amino acid release in skeletal muscle cells. IL 1, IL 6 and TNF reduce liver protein biosynthesis and protein production focuses on acute phase proteins (CRP, alpha-1-antitrypsine) instead of carrier proteins (i.e. albumin). TNF is partially responsible for high plasma triglyceride levels by inhibiting lipoproteinlipase on endothelial cell membranes and therefore the triglyceride release from VLDL.

Consequently, therapeutical strategies during the flow phase therefore focus on metabolic support and not on maintaining body mass until stress factors can be reduced. Nutritional therapy should be adapted to the utilization capacity of the patient. A relapse into the ebb phase is possible at any point in time (disturbed organ function, hemodynamic instability).

The organism can only enter a state of reparation after all stress-inducing factors have been eliminated. Only then do physiological neuro- endocrine circumstances allow an undisturbed substrate metabolism. A positive energy and nitrogen balance can be set as a therapeutical goal. In most cases patients do not reach the reparative phase until after having been discharged from ICU.

3.6.1. Enteral Versus Parenteral Nutrition

While “vital” organ function is the main focus in intensive care little attention is paid to intestine function. At the same time the intestine is substantially involved in post-aggression metabolism and as the "motor of sepsis" [77,120]. Motility, absorption and immunological functions are altered with in part major consequences for the entire organism. A permeability disturbance of the intestinal barrier with a resulting translocation of bacteria and/or bacterial components (endotoxins, peptidoglykanes) from the intestine is considered an important initiator of the systemic inflammation syndrome (SIRS), from which in consequence a multi-organ failure can develop. As possible factors initiating intestine damage ischemia/ reperfusion, inflammation, changed bacterial flora, malnutrition as well as hyperalimentation are regarded as aspects of the "gut injury hypothesis" [53,103,128]. After numerous positive animal experiments a correlation could be established between the bacterial translocation and the incidence of septic complications which could also be documented in humans [53,103].

Which factors are relevant for enteral nutrition in comparison to parenteral nutrition regarding the prevention of intestine-associated septic complications? On the one hand, the danger of bacterial translocation from the intestine is lower using enteral rather than parenteral nutrition [53,103]. Enteral nutrition physiologically stimulates peristalsis and can prevent intestine paralysis, frequently induced by abdominal surgery, septic complications or anesthetics and sedatives. In addition, lack of enteral food intake leads to a decrease of intestine mass, vili height and intestine-associated lymphatic system function. Enteral nutrition as opposed to total parenteral nutrition contributes to the maintenance of biliary IgA secretion. As preservation of an intact intestinal mucosal barrier is one goal of the nutritional therapy, early post-operative or post-traumatic enteral nutrition is of crucial importance.

Certain studies from the late 80ies raised concerns that TPN might increase infectious complications and induce a fatty liver in critically ill patients [38,79]. A critical review of the data suggests that, in humans, TPN does not cause mucosal atrophy or increase bacterial translocation [70] and that increased sepsis with TPN can be ascribed to overfeeding [63]. Accordingly, Wolfe concluded that clinical phenomena, such as existing liver disease, renal failure, and abdominal sepsis, rather than the administration of TPN had a predominant effect on liver histopathology [136]. Heyland performed a meta-analysis of 26 randomised controlled trials in which TPN was compared with standard care [63]. These trials included 2211 patients undergoing surgery, patients with burns, patients with pancreatitis, and patients in intensive care units. Although TPN did not reduce the overall mortality and morbidity, a significantly reduced morbidity was found in malnourished patients. Since malnutrition increases the risk of morbidity in hospitalised patients [101], and nutritional goals are reached earlier with TPN (day 1 vs. day 4) [13], the parenteral route seems to be feasible to prevent underfeeding in the early course of clinical nutrition when gastrointestinal problems are present [13,63,70,101,103,113].

The two main factors contributing to the duration of hospitalization in a multifactor-regression calculation were the amount of omega-6 FA (+1.6d/ 100g) and a delay of intravenous nutritional support (+1.42d/ day of TPN-delay) (figure 28a). In accordance with other studies recent meta analyses, and derived guidelines [13,62] we were able to show furthermore that following an initial phase of supportive TPN early enteral feeding resulted in a significant reduction in hospital stay [80] (figure 28c). Each 24-hour delay of enteral feeding further extended hospital stay by 0.58 days. Thus, optimizing the nutrition management to instant i.v.-support on admission to ICU and starting enteral nutrition as early as possible may save up to 2 days of hospitalization per day of adequate nutritional support. Hyperalimentation on the contrary had a negative impact on the patients' condition, because high blood glucose levels extended hospital stay by 0.53 days per 10 mg/dl. This observation backs the concept of strict avoidance of hyperalimentation as well as tight control of blood glucose levels [128].

An interesting aspect was the fact that early enteral feeding tended to be specifically delayed if high calorie parenteral diets had previously been applied (figure 28b). This may on the one hand be explained by a perhaps difficult initiation of enteral feeding resulting in a negative patient selection. On the other hand it cannot be ruled out that the intensive care staff just did not discontinue effective and sufficient parenteral feeding. Early enteral support is a key factor in the improvement of survival as depicted in figure 28d. Therefore, these results underscore the necessity to early initiate enteral feeding even if parenteral feeding is in line with metabolic demand. The decision to begin enteral feeding should be made on a daily basis and hyperalimentation in particular should be avoided.

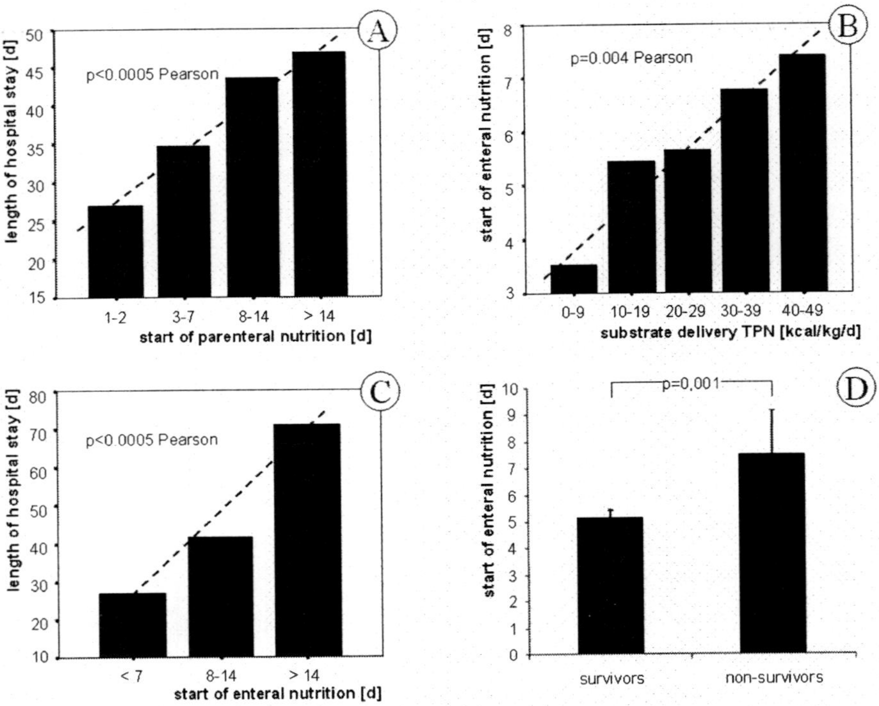

Figure 28. Impact of the management of enteral and parenteral nutrition in 661 patients. A) Correlation between the start of TPN after ICU admission and the length of hospital stay. Each day of postponement of initial i.v. nutritional support delays hospital discharge by 1.42 days. B) Correlation between start of enteral nutrition and daily parenteral substrate delivery. C) Correlation between the onset enteral nutrition and the length of hospital stay. Each day of postponement of enteral nutrition delays hospital discharge by 2.0 days. D) Early enteral nutrition was associated with higher survival rates.

Nutritional goals have changed over the last two decades from immunosuppressant hyperalimentation to more reasonable objectives [128], and the quality of intravenous lipid emulsions evolved likewise [3]. TPN is an equally effective alternative to EN when a risk of malnutrition is present and EN is not tolerated or when gut failure is present [38,79].

According to recent studies an effective coverage of metabolic demands must be achieved in severely ill patients from the first day on [13,80]. Bower and coworkers combined TPN with enteral nutrition in critically ill patients with a mean SAPS II score of 42. They observed, that the described nutritional goal of 25kcal/kg/d could not be achieved solely via the enteral route until day seven, whereas an i.v.-infusion of missing enteral calories ascertained that all patients in the combined EN/TPN group reached the nutritional goal from day one onwards [13]. Patients in the enteral group, thus, received an average caloric load of 13.7/kg per day over the study period as opposed to the combined group who obtained 25 kcal/d, resulting in an earlier hospital discharge (34 vs. 31 days) in that group.

In view of the metabolic kinetics of exogenously taken omega-3 fatty acids, differences between oral and parenteral administration are under discussion. While oral intake leads to the inclusion of omega-3 FA in cellular membranes after a diet of several days' duration, after parenteral administration omega-3 FA are incorporated and metabolized even faster [95]. This observation is due to the fact, that local cellular lipid uptake mechanisms are bypassed by intravenous application, which overcomes kinetics and the extent of dietary application by order of magnitude [48].

The amount of omega-3 fatty acids in the membrane phospholipids of leukocytes and erythrocytes rose as early as during the first infusion day in healthy volunteers who received 10% of their fat intake in form of fish oil intravenously [24]. In patients after major abdominal surgery, too, a rapid rise in EPA (the effective omega-3 fatty acid) in plasma and blood cells occurred as early as three days after the start of Omegaven infusion [49], whereas after oral administration no noticeable effect could be shown within this period [44,95].

Enteral nutrition has significant advantages for the preservation of the intestinal and metabolic function as well as for survival [62]. Thus, the main target of modern nutrition therapy is to offer patients a nutrition specially adapted to metabolic demands (substrate guided, overflow limited). Accordingly, today's standard of care in severely ill patients, as investigated in our studies, is early (12h post trauma/ surgery) *enteral* feeding e.g. by intraoperatively placed small bowel catheters [62] or other multimodal concepts [59,72]. Parenteral nutrition may be chosen during episodes of insufficient or impaired intestinal transport and mucosal uptake function, to guarantee better bioavailability of the administered nutrients. Moreover, additional parenteral administration of nutrients during insufficient enteral nutrition may facilitate the achievement of caloric nutritional objectives. The latter concept may even be optimized when reasonable caloric goals (15-25 kcal/kg/d) are consistently combined with a tight control of blood glucose with insulin.

"If the gut works, use it! "

3.6.2. Indications for Enteral / Parenteral Nutrition

If stable metabolic and hemodynamics are present and if the gastrointestinal tract is functionally intact enteral nutrition is the physiological, most effective nutritive therapy with the lowest risk factor. A naso-jejunal tube with partial parenteral supplementation should be used if gastrointestinal function is only partially intact.

contraindications for enteral nutrition (EN)	
Absolute	• Patients with marginal protective reflexes (in danger of aspiration when non- intubated) • Obstructive and paralytical ileus • Gastrointestinal bleeding • Acute necrotising pancreatitis • Metabolic coma • All shock forms and severe hemodynamic instability • Planned surgery or extubation within 6 hrs
Relative	• Frequent nausea and vomiting • Gastral reflux (>1 liter /day)

Indications for total parenteral nutrition (TPN)	
Absolute	Disturbances of gastrointestinal nutrition uptake, • Extensive small bowel resections • Acute phase of chronic enterocolitis, • Radiation-induced enteritis • Recurring diarrhoea (>3 times 300 ml/ day), • Recurring vomiting (>1 liter/ day), • Paralytic and obstructive ileus • Acute hemorrhagic- necrotizing pancreatitis, • High dose chemotherapy, radiation therapy, after bone marrow transplantation • Severe malnutrition due to pre-operative intestinal malfunction (begin parenteral nutrition post-operatively).
TPN possible	• Surgery of injuries of the gastro-intestinal system • Enterocutane fistula • Inflammatory bowel disease • Hyperemesis gravidarum • Supplementation of enteral nutrition
Contra-indications	• Intact gastrointestinal system • Shock with hemodynamic instability • Metabolic derailment (massive metabolic acidosis, diabetic coma) • Severe coagulation disorders (DIC IV°).

3.6.3. Immunonutrition/ Pharmaconutrition

Nutrition solutions enriched with special substances that have favorable effects on the immune system are called immunonutrition or, recently, even pharmaconutrition. The strict separation between nutritive therapy and pharmacotherapy therefore is increasingly disappearing. While aliments are considered substances which maintain nutritive or metabolic processes of the organism, drugs are chemical substances which can improve a pathophysiological condition. Immunonutrition or pharmaconutrition decreases the incidence and extent of septic complications (i.e. multiorgan failure) by means of their dual function [1]. By reducing length of hospital stay and antibiotic therapy a net cost saving is possible despite higher expenditures for the substances involved [1,15]. At present a mixture of nucleotides, arginine and omega-3 FA is commonly used. Since pharmaconutritients are important as membrane components and modulators of biochemical processes, the goal of an optimized nutritional therapy should be to combine pharmacological, energetic and essential features of different substrates in an optimal way. To evaluate the multitude of work with differential outcome on immunonutrition in recent years [39] meta-analyses have been performed [15,64,66]. As a matter of fact, by using such mixtures the effect of a single component cannot be identified, complicating any improvement of such solutions.

Firm recommendations regarding nutrition therapy were formulated during a consensus conference in May 2001, when existing evidence for beneficial effects of immunonutrition and respective target groups was presented [1]. These recommendations were backed up by the meta-analysis done by Heyland and others who examined 326 studies involving 2419 patients [64]. This analysis showed a slight, but non-significant reduction of mortality by immunonutrition. The risk of post-operative infectious complications was significantly lower in the immunonutrition group (RR 0.53; CI 95%: 0.42-0.68). The length of hospital stay was significantly reduced both for post-operative and critically ill patients by an average of 3.3 days. On the basis of this differentiated evaluation recommendations for immunonutrition were given (Grade A recommendations with level I evidence).

Patients who definitely (evidence-based medicine) benefit from immunonutrition therapy are therefore those with elective gastro-intestinal surgery, in particular with preexisting malnutrition (albumin < 35 g/l), and patients with multiple trauma and / or blunt or penetrating torso trauma (Injury severity score ≥ 18).

Patients who are likely to profit from immunonutritive therapy are: patients with elective aortal surgery (with COPD or foreseeable pulmonary therapy), head and neck surgery with pre- existing malnutrition, cerebral trauma with GCS < 8 and pathological CT, burns > 30%, grade 3 und ventilator dependent patients with a risk of non-septic infections.

No evidence of any beneficial effect was documented for patients who are expected to resume an oral *ad libitum* diet within five days, for those with short stay monitoring and with incomplete resuscitation and splanchnic hypoperfusion. Accordingly, recent data from Bertholini [16] questioned the concept of immunonutrition in critically ill patients, since a higher mortality rate in patients receiving enteral immunonutrition was observed. The editorial on this article by Heyland [65] stated: "*... immune-modulating nutrients (for example, arginine) that enhance cytokine release and/or increase nitric oxide production may do more harm than good in critically ill patients with sepsis or any population characterized by an over-amplified inflammatory response, arginine-containing immune-enhancing diets should not be used in patients with sepsis ...*" Thus, one might conclude that the multitude of beneficial effects reported for immune-enhanced nutritional solutions is attributable to the other constituents, namely omega-3 FA and nucleotides.

Considering the timing of enteral immunonutrition it should at best commence 5-7 days pre-operatively, or else as soon as possible post-operatively, e.g. by naso-gastral or jejunal tube if necessary with 1.200-1.500 ml/day. Therapy should last for at least 5-10 days, or as long as infectious complications are to be expected (CRP↓, Prealbumin↑).

Patients after massive trauma, large abdominal operations, or systemic inflammation show a major metabolic and immunological derailment (hyperinflammation/immunparalysis). In these cases a metabolism-orientated therapy combined with immunonutritive therapy [1,15,39,64,66,103,114] is beneficial. Depending on the severity of the underlying illness energy input may possibly be reduced to a minimum need ("metabolic support") or must even be discontinued in severe septic shock (ebb phase). Individual organ failure does not, however, exclude enteral or parenteral substitution as long as normal utilization can be expected (triglycerides <3-4mmol/l; <260-350g/dl).

3.7. References

[1] (2001) Proceedings from Summit on Immune-Enhancing Enteral Therapy. May 25-26, 2000, San Diego, California, USA. *JPEN J.Parenter.Enteral Nutr.* 25:S1-63.

[2] Abraham E., Anzueto A., Gutierrez G., Tessler S., San Pedro G., Wunderink R., Dal Nogare A., Nasraway S., Berman S., Cooney R., Levy H., Baughman R., Rumbak M., Light R. B., Poole L., Allred R., Constant J., Pennington J., Porter S. (1998) Double-blind randomised controlled trial of monoclonal antibody to human tumour necrosis factor in treatment of septic shock. NORASEPT II Study Group. *Lancet* 351:929-933.

[3] Adolph M. (1999) Lipid emulsions in parenteral nutrition. *Ann.Nutr.Metab* 43:1-13.

[4] Alexander J. W.Gottschlich M. M. (1990) Nutritional immunomodulation in burn patients. *Crit Care Med.* 18:S149-S153.

[5] Ayala A.Chaudry I. H. (1996) Immune dysfunction in murine polymicrobial sepsis: mediators, macrophages, lymphocytes and apoptosis. *Shock* 6 Suppl 1:S27-S38.

[6] Bach R. R. (1988) Initiation of coagulation by tissue factor. *CRC Crit Rev.Biochem.* 23:339-368.

[7] Baker S. P., O'Neill B., Haddon W., Jr., Long W. B. (1974) The injury severity score: a method for describing patients with multiple injuries and evaluating emergency care. *J.Trauma* 14:187-196.

[8] Barber M. D., McMillan D. C., Preston T., Ross J. A., Fearon K. C. (2000) Metabolic response to feeding in weight-losing pancreatic cancer patients and its modulation by a fish-oil-enriched nutritional supplement. *Clin.Sci.(*Lond) 98:389-399.

[9] Barber M. D., Ross J. A., Preston T., Shenkin A., Fearon K. C. (1999) Fish oil-enriched nutritional supplement attenuates progression of the acute phase response in weight-losing patients with advanced pancreatic cancer. *J.Nutr.* 129:1120-1125.

[10] Barber M. D., Ross J. A., Voss A. C., Tisdale M. J., Fearon K. C. (1999) The effect of an oral nutritional supplement enriched with fish oil on weight-loss in patients with pancreatic cancer. *Br.J.Cancer* 81:80-86.

[11] Barton R. G., Wells C. L., Carlson A., Singh R., Sullivan J. J., Cerra F. B. (1991) Dietary omega-3 fatty acids decrease mortality and Kupffer cell prostaglandin E2 production in a rat model of chronic sepsis. *J.Trauma* 31:768-773.

[12] Bastian L., Weimann A., Bischoff W., Meier P. N., Grotz M., Stan C., Regel G. (1998) [Clinical effects of supplemental enteral nutrition solution in severe polytrauma]. *Unfallchirurg* 101:105-114.

[13] Bauer P., Charpentier C., Bouchet C., Nace L., Raffy F., Gaconnet N. (2000) Parenteral with enteral nutrition in the critically ill. *Intensive Care Med.* 26:893-900.

[14] Baumann H.Gauldie J. (1994) The acute phase response. *Immunol.Today* 15:74-80.

[15] Beale R. J., Bryg D. J., Bihari D. J. (1999) Immunonutrition in the critically ill: a systematic review of clinical outcome. *Crit Care Med.* 27:2799-2805.

[16] Bertolini G., Iapichino G., Radrizzani D., Facchini R., Simini B., Bruzzone P., Zanforlin G., Tognoni G. (2003) Early enteral immunonutrition in patients with severe sepsis: results of an interim analysis of a randomized multicentre clinical trial. *Intensive Care Med.* 29:834-840.

[17] Bone R. C. (1996) Sir Isaac Newton, sepsis, SIRS, and CARS. *Crit Care Med.* 24:1125-1128.

[18] Bone R. C. (1996) Toward a theory regarding the pathogenesis of the systemic inflammatory response syndrome: what we do and do not know about cytokine regulation. *Crit Care Med.* 24:163-172.

[19] Brain S. D., Camp R. D., Dowd P. M., Black A. K., Woollard P. M., Mallet A. I., Greaves M. W. (1982) Psoriasis and leukotriene B4. *Lancet* 2:762-763.

[20] Breil I., Koch T., Heller A., Schlotzer E., Grunert A., van Ackern K., Neuhof H. (1996) Alteration of n-3 fatty acid composition in lung tissue after short-term infusion of fish oil emulsion attenuates inflammatory vascular reaction. *Crit Care Med.* 24:1893-1902.

[21] Calder P. C. (1996) Can n-3 polyunsaturated fatty acids be used as immunomodulatory agents? *Biochem.Soc.Trans.* 24:211-220.

[22] Calder P. C. (1996) Effects of fatty acids and dietary lipids on cells of the immune system. *Proc.Nutr.Soc.* 55:127-150.

[23] Calder P. C., Yaqoob P., Thies F., Wallace F. A., Miles E. A. (2002) Fatty acids and lymphocyte functions. *Br.J.Nutr.* 87 Suppl 1:S31-S48.

[24] Carpentier Y. A., Simoens C., Siderova V., el Nakadi, I, Vanweyenberg V., Eggerickx D., Deckelbaum R. J. (1997) Recent developments in lipid emulsions: relevance to intensive care. *Nutrition* 13:73S-78S.

[25] Caygill C. P., Charlett A., Hill M. J. (1996) Fat, fish, fish oil and cancer. *Br.J.Cancer* 74:159-164.

[26] Chandrasekar B.Fernandes G. (1994) Decreased pro-inflammatory cytokines and increased antioxidant enzyme gene expression by omega-3 lipids in murine lupus nephritis. *Biochem.Biophys.Res.Commun.* 200:893-898.

[27] Dhainaut J. F., Tenaillon A., Le Tulzo Y., Schlemmer B., Solet J. P., Wolff M., Holzapfel L., Zeni F., Dreyfuss D., Mira J. P., . (1994) Platelet-activating factor receptor antagonist BN 52021 in the treatment of severe sepsis: a randomized, double-blind, placebo-controlled, multicenter clinical trial. BN 52021 Sepsis Study Group. *Crit Care Med.* 22:1720-1728.

[28] Dyerberg J.Bang H. O. (1995) Haemostatic function and platelet polyunsaturated fatty acids in Eskimos. 1979. *Nutrition* 11:475-

[29] Dyerberg J., Bang H. O., Hjorne N. (1975) Fatty acid composition of the plasma lipids in Greenland Eskimos. *Am.J.Clin.Nutr.* 28:958-966.

[30] Dyerberg J., Bang H. O., Stoffersen E., Moncada S., Vane J. R. (1978) Eicosapentaenoic acid and prevention of thrombosis and atherosclerosis? *Lancet* 2:117-119.

[31] Elgert K. D., Alleva D. G., Mullins D. W. (1998) Tumor-induced immune dysfunction: the macrophage connection. *J.Leukoc.Biol.* 64:275-290.

[32] Endres S., Ghorbani R., Kelley V. E., Georgilis K., Lonnemann G., van der Meer J. W., Cannon J. G., Rogers T. S., Klempner M. S., Weber P. C., . (1989) The effect of dietary supplementation with n-3 polyunsaturated fatty acids on the synthesis of interleukin-1 and tumor necrosis factor by mononuclear cells. *N.Engl.J.Med.* 320:265-271.

[33] Ertel W., Morrison M. H., Ayala A., Chaudry I. H. (1993) Modulation of macrophage membrane phospholipids by n-3 polyunsaturated fatty acids increases interleukin 1 release and prevents suppression of cellular immunity following hemorrhagic shock. *Arch.Surg.* 128:15-20.

[34] Faist E., Hartl W. H., Baue A. E. (1994) [Immune mechanisms of post-traumatic hyperinflammation and sepsis]. *Immun.Infekt.* 22:203-213.

[35] Falconer J. S., Fearon K. C., Ross J. A., Elton R., Wigmore S. J., Garden O. J., Carter D. C. (1995) Acute-phase protein response and survival duration of patients with pancreatic cancer. *Cancer* 75:2077-2082.

[36] Fearon K. C. H. (2002) The anticancer and anticachectic effects of n-3 fatty acids. *Clin Nutr* 21:69-73.

[37] Friedman G., Silva E., Vincent J. L. (1998) Has the mortality of septic shock changed with time. *Crit Care Med.* 26:2078-2086.

[38] Gadek J. E., DeMichele S. J., Karlstad M. D., Pacht E. R., Donahoe M., Albertson T. E., Van Hoozen C., Wennberg A. K., Nelson J. L., Noursalehi M. (1999) Effect of enteral feeding with eicosapentaenoic acid, gamma-linolenic acid, and antioxidants in patients with acute respiratory distress syndrome. Enteral Nutrition in ARDS Study Group. *Crit Care Med.* 27:1409-1420.

[39] Galban C., Montejo J. C., Mesejo A., Marco P., Celaya S., Sanchez-Segura J. M., Farre M., Bryg D. J. (2000) An immune-enhancing enteral diet reduces mortality rate and episodes of bacteremia in septic intensive care unit patients. *Crit Care Med.* 28:643-648.

[40] Geusens P., Wouters C., Nijs J., Jiang Y., Dequeker J. (1994) Long-term effect of omega-3 fatty acid supplementation in active rheumatoid arthritis. A 12-month, double-blind, controlled study. *Arthritis Rheum.* 37:824-829.

[41] Grecu I, Mirea L, Grintescu I (2003) Parenteral fish oil supplementation in patients with abdominal sepsis. *Clin Nutr* 22:23-

[42] Grimm H., Tibell A., Norrlind B., Blecher C., Wilker S., Schwemmle K. (1994) Immunoregulation by parenteral lipids: impact of the n-3 to n-6 fatty acid ratio. *JPEN J.Parenter.Enteral Nutr.* 18:417-421.

[43] Grimm H., Tibell A., Norrlind B., Schott J., Bohle R. M., Papavassilis C., Fuhrer D., Mayer K., Grimminger F. (1995) [Immunosuppressive effect of parenteral fat emulsions in defined immunostimulation]. *Infusionsther.Transfusionsmed.* 22:110-116.

[44] Grimminger F., Fuhrer D., Papavassilis C., Schlotzer E., Mayer K., Heuer K. U., Kiss L., Walmrath D., Piberhofer S., Lubbecke F., . (1993) Influence of intravenous n-3

lipid supplementation on fatty acid profiles and lipid mediator generation in a patient with severe ulcerative colitis. *Eur.J.Clin.Invest* 23:706-715.

[45] Grimminger F., Mayer K., Kramer H. J., Stevens J., Walmrath D., Seeger W. (1993) Differential vasoconstrictor potencies of free fatty acids in the lung vasculature: 2-versus 3-series prostanoid generation. *J.Pharmacol.Exp.Ther.* 267:259-265.

[46] Grimminger F., Mayer K., Walmrath D., Schlotzer E., Seeger W. (1995) Omega-3-fatty acids and inflammatory diseases. In: Cynober, L., Fürst, P., and Lawin, P. (Hrsg.) Pharmacological Nutrition Immune Nutrition, Zuckerschwerdt. *Aufl.* 116-121.

[47] Grimminger F., Mayser P., Papavassilis C., Thomas M., Schlotzer E., Heuer K. U., Fuhrer D., Hinsch K. D., Walmrath D., Schill W. B., . (1993) A double-blind, randomized, placebo-controlled trial of n-3 fatty acid based lipid infusion in acute, extended guttate psoriasis. Rapid improvement of clinical manifestations and changes in neutrophil leukotriene profile. *Clin.Investig.* 71:634-643.

[48] Grimminger F., Seeger W., Mayer K. (2002) Use of n-3 fatty acid-containing lipid emulsions in the intensive care unit environment: the clinician's view. *Clin Nutr* 21:21-27.

[49] Hailer S., Matthias M., Wolf S., Jauch K. W., Wolfram G. (2001) Influence of fish oil containing emulsions on plasma lipids and blood cell membranes in patients after major abdominal surgery. *Clin Nutr* 20:40-41.

[50] Hamawy K. J., Moldawer L. L., Georgieff M., Valicenti A. J., Babayan V. K., Bistrian B. R., Blackburn G. L. (1985) The Henry M. Vars Award. The effect of lipid emulsions on reticuloendothelial system function in the injured animal. *JPEN J.Parenter.Enteral Nutr.* 9:559-565.

[51] MacLean C. H., Newberry S. J., Mojica W. A., Khanna P, Issa A. M., Suttorp M. J., Lim Y. W., Traina S. B., Hilton L, Garland R, Morton S. C. (2006) Effects of omega-3 fatty acids on cancer risk: a systematic review. *JAMA.* 295(4):403-15.

[52] Hartert H. H. (1981) Resonance-thrombography, theoretical and practical elements. *Biorheology* 18:693-701.

[53] Hawker F. H. (2000) How to feed patients with sepsis. *Curr.Opin.Crit Care* 6:247-252.

[54] Hayashi N., Tashiro T., Yamamori H., Takagi K., Morishima Y., Otsubo Y., Sugiura T., Furukawa K., Nitta H., Nakajima N., Suzuki N., Ito I. (1998) Effects of intravenous omega-3 and omega-6 fat emulsion on cytokine production and delayed type hypersensitivity in burned rats receiving total parenteral nutrition. *JPEN J.Parenter.Enteral Nutr.* 22:363-367.

[55] Heller A., Koch T., Schmeck J., van Ackern K. (1998) Lipid mediators in inflammatory disorders. *Drugs* 55:487-496.

[56] Heller A. R. (1998) Einfluß einer Omega-3-Lipidlösung auf die inflammatorische Gefäßantwort: Untersuchungen am Modell der isoliert perfundierten Kaninchenlunge. Doctoral Thesis at the Department of Internal Medicine, Medical School University of Giessen, Germany

[57] Heller AR, Fischer S, Roessel T, Gottschlich B, Ragaller M, Tiebel O, Menschikowski M, Zimmermann T, Albrecht DM, Koch T (2001) Immunonutritional aspects of parenteral fish oil supplementation after major abdominal surgery. *Crit Care Med.* 29:A127-

[58] Heller A. R., Groth G., Heller S. C., Breitkreutz R., Nebe T., Quintel M., Koch T. (2001) N-acetylcysteine reduces respiratory burst but augments neutrophil phagocytosis in intensive care unit patients. *Crit Care Med.* 29:272-276.

[59] Heller A. R., Litz R. J., Djonlagic I., Manseck A., Koch T., Wirth M. P., Albrecht D. M. (2000) [Combined anesthesia with epidural catheter. A retrospective analysis of the perioperative course in patients undergoing radical prostatectomy]. *Anaesthesist* 49:949-959.

[60] Heller A. R., Rössel T., Gottschlich B., Tiebel O., Menschikowski M., Litz R. J., Zimmermann T., Koch T. (2004) Omega-3 fatty acids improve liver and pancreas function in postoperative cancer patients. *Int.J.Cance*r 111:611-616.

[61] Heller A. R., Rössler S., Litz R. J., Stehr S. N., Heller S. C., Koch T. (2006) Omega-3 fatty acids improve the diagnosis- related clinical outcome. *Crit Care Med.* 38 (4):pp

[62] Heyland D. K., Dhaliwal R., Drover J. W., Gramlich L., Dodek P. (2003) Canadian clinical practice guidelines for nutrition support in mechanically ventilated, critically ill adult patients. *JPEN J.Parenter.Enteral Nutr*. 27:355-373.

[63] Heyland D. K., MacDonald S., Keefe L., Drover J. W. (1998) Total parenteral nutrition in the critically ill patient: a meta-analysis. *JAMA* 280:2013-2019.

[64] Heyland D. K., Novak F., Drover J. W., Jain M., Su X., Suchner U. (2001) Should immunonutrition become routine in critically ill patients? A systematic review of the evidence. *JAMA* 286:944-953.

[65] Heyland D. K.Samis A. (2003) Does immunonutrition in patients with sepsis do more harm than good? *Intensive Care Med.* 29:669-671.

[66] Heys S. D., Walker L. G., Smith I., Eremin O. (1999) Enteral nutritional supplementation with key nutrients in patients with critical illness and cancer: a meta-analysis of randomized controlled clinical trials. *Ann.Surg*. 229:467-477.

[67] Hosotsubo K. K., Nishimura M., Nishimura S. (2000) Hyperbilirubinaemia after major thoracic surgery: comparison between open-heart surgery and oesophagectomy. *Crit Care* 4:180-187.

[68] Hower R, Kiefer B, Marzi I, Buehren V, Harbauer G, Tretz O (1990) Lobular distribution and activation of hepatic macrophages following hemorrhagic shock in the rat. *Circ Shock* 31:52.

[69] Hwang TL, Huang YS, Huang YC, Yang YM (2000) The prevention of apoptotic changes of hepatocytes in rats of sepsis after fed with immunomodulational diet. Proceedings of the 6th PENSA Congress

[70] Jeejeebhoy K. N. (2001) Total parenteral nutrition: potion or poison? *Am.J.Clin.Nutr.* 74:160-163.

[71] Johnson J. A., III, Griswold J. A., Muakkassa F. F. (1993) Essential fatty acids influence survival in sepsis. J.Trauma 35:128-131.

[72] Kehlet H.Wilmore D. W. (2002) Multimodal strategies to improve surgical outcome. *Am.J.Surg*. 183:630-641.

[73] Kelbel I., Koch T., Prechtl A., Heller A., Schlotzer E., Schiefer G., Neuhof H. (1999) Effects of Parenteral Application of Fish Oil versus Soy Oil Emulsions on Bacterial Clearance functions. *Infusionsther.Transfusionsmed.* 26:226-232.

[74] Kelbel I., Wagner F., Wiedeck-Suger H, Kelbel M, Weiss M, Schneider M, Grünert A, Hartung T, Georgieff M (2002) Effects of n-3 fatty acids on immune function: A double- blind, randomized trial of fish oil based infusion in postoperative patients. *Clin Nutr* 21:P39-

[75] Kinsella J. E., Lokesh B., Broughton S., Whelan J. (1990) Dietary polyunsaturated fatty acids and eicosanoids: potential effects on the modulation of inflammatory and immune cells: an overview. *Nutrition* 6:24-44.

[76] Knapp H. R. (1997) Dietary fatty acids in human thrombosis and hemostasis. *Am.J.Clin.Nutr.* 65:1687S-1698S.

[77] Knisely M. H., Cowley R. A., Hawthorne I., Garris D. (1970) Separation of shock types. Experimental and clinical separation of hypovolemic and septic shock. *Angiology* 21:728-744.

[78] Koch T., Duncker H. P., Klein A., Neuhof H., van Ackern K. (1993) Effects of omega-3-fatty acids on pulmonary vascular reaction: A therapeutical approach in citical illness. *Clin Intens Care* 4:10-

[79] Koch T., Duncker H. P., Klein A., Schlotzer E., Peskar B. M., van Ackern K., Neuhof H. (1993) Modulation of pulmonary vascular resistance and edema formation by short-term infusion of a 10% fish oil emulsion. Infusionsther.*Transfusionsmed.* 20:291-300.

[80] Koch T.Heller A. (2005) Outcome-Effects of parenteral nutrition with omega-3 fatty acids - a multicenter observation in 661 patients. *Aktuel.Ernaehr.Med.* 30:15-22.

[81] Koch T., Heller A., Breil I., van Ackern K., Neuhof H. (1995) Alterations of pulmonary capillary filtration and leukotriene synthesis due to infusion of a lipid emulsion enriched with Omega-3-fatty acids. *Clin Intens Care* 6:112-120.

[82] Kremer J. M., Lawrence D. A., Petrillo G. F., Litts L. L., Mullaly P. M., Rynes R. I., Stocker R. P., Parhami N., Greenstein N. S., Fuchs B. R., . (1995) Effects of high-dose fish oil on rheumatoid arthritis after stopping nonsteroidal antiinflammatory drugs. Clinical and immune correlates. *Arthritis Rheum.* 38:1107-1114.

[83] Lanier L. L., Le A. M., Civin C. I., Loken M. R., Phillips J. H. (1986) The relationship of CD16 (Leu-11) and Leu-19 (NKH-1) antigen expression on human peripheral blood NK cells and cytotoxic T lymphocytes. *J.Immunol.* 136:4480-4486.

[84] Le Gall, Jr., Lemeshow S., Saulnier F. (1993) A new Simplified Acute Physiology Score (SAPS II) based on a European/North American multicenter study. *JAMA* 270:2957-2963.

[85] Lehr H. A., Hubner C., Finckh B., Nolte D., Beisiegel U., Kohlschutter A., Messmer K. (1991) Dietary fish oil reduces leukocyte/endothelium interaction following systemic administration of oxidatively modified low density lipoprotein. *Circulation* 84:1725-1731.

[86] Levy M. M., Fink M. P., Marshall J. C., Abraham E., Angus D., Cook D., Cohen J., Opal S. M., Vincent J. L., Ramsay G. (2003) 2001 SCCM/ESICM/ACCP/ATS/SIS International Sepsis Definitions Conference. *Crit Care Med.* 31:1250-1256.

[87] Levy M. M., Pronovost P. J., Dellinger R. P., Townsend S., Resar R. K., Clemmer T. P., Ramsay G. (2004) Sepsis change bundles: converting guidelines into meaningful change in behavior and clinical outcome. *Crit Care Med.* 32:S595-S597.

[88] Lobos E. A., Sharon P., Stenson W. F. (1987) Chemotactic activity in inflammatory bowel disease. Role of leukotriene B4. *Dig.Dis.Sci.* 32:1380-1388.

[89] Mahoney E. M., Hamill A. L., Scott W. A., Cohn Z. A. (1977) Response of endocytosis to altered fatty acyl composition of macrophage phospholipids. *Proc.Natl.Acad.Sci.*U.S.A 74:4895-4899.

[90] Marciniak R., Majewski P., Biczysko M., Banasiewicz T., Wozniak A., Drews M. (2004) Effects of gastrectomy or colectomy on liver metabolism and liver morphology in an experimental rat model. *Med.Sci.Monit.* 10:BR34-BR40.

[91] Mayer K., Fegbeutel C., Hattar K., Sibelius U., Kramer H. J., Heuer K. U., Temmesfeld-Wollbruck B., Gokorsch S., Grimminger F., Seeger W. (2003) Omega-3 vs. omega-6 lipid emulsions exert differential influence on neutrophils in septic shock patients: impact on plasma fatty acids and lipid mediator generation. *Intensive Care Med.* 29:1472-1481.

[92] Mayer K., Gokorsch S., Fegbeutel C., Hattar K., Rosseau S., Walmrath D., Seeger W., Grimminger F. (2003) Parenteral nutrition with fish oil modulates cytokine response in patients with sepsis. *Am.J.Respir.Crit Care Med.* 167:1321-1328.

[93] Mayer K., Grimm H., Grimminger F., Seeger W. (2002) Parenteral nutrition with n-3 lipids in sepsis. *Br.J.Nutr.* 87 Suppl 1:S69-S75.

[94] Mayer K., Meyer S., Reinholz-Muhly M., Maus U., Merfels M., Lohmeyer J., Grimminger F., Seeger W. (2003) Short-time infusion of fish oil-based lipid emulsions, approved for parenteral nutrition, reduces monocyte proinflammatory cytokine generation and adhesive interaction with endothelium in humans. *J.Immunol.* 171:4837-4843.

[95] Mayser P., Mayer K., Mahloudjian M., Benzing S., Kramer H. J., Schill W. B., Seeger W., Grimminger F. (2002) A double-blind, randomized, placebo-controlled trial of n-3 versus n-6 fatty acid-based lipid infusion in atopic dermatitis. *JPEN J.Parenter.Enteral Nutr* 26:151-158.

[96] Mischke R. (2000) Sensitivity of the reaction time of the resonance thrombogram for factor VIII:C and factor IX deficiencies in the blood of dogs with haemophilia A or B. *Haemophilia.* 6:575-580.

[97] Mitropoulos K. A., Martin J. C., Reeves B. E., Esnouf M. P. (1989) The activation of the contact phase of coagulation by physiologic surfaces in plasma: the effect of large negatively charged liposomal vesicles. *Blood* 73:1525-1533.

[98] Moldawer L. L.Copeland E. M., III (1997) Proinflammatory cytokines, nutritional support, and the cachexia syndrome: interactions and therapeutic options. *Cancer* 79:1828-1839.

[99] Molvig J., Pociot F., Worsaae H., Wogensen L. D., Baek L., Christensen P., Mandrup-Poulsen T., Andersen K., Madsen P., Dyerberg J., . (1991) Dietary supplementation with omega-3-polyunsaturated fatty acids decreases mononuclear cell proliferation and interleukin-1 beta content but not monokine secretion in healthy and insulin-dependent diabetic individuals. *Scand.J.Immunol.* 34:399-410.

[100] Mosmann T. R.Sad S. (1996) The expanding universe of T-cell subsets: Th1, Th2 and more. *Immunol.Today* 17:138-146.

[101] Naber T. H., Schermer T., de Bree A., Nusteling K., Eggink L., Kruimel J. W., Bakkeren J., van Heereveld H., Katan M. B. (1997) Prevalence of malnutrition in nonsurgical hospitalized patients and its association with disease complications. *Am.J.Clin Nutr* 66:1232-1239.

[102] Narayanan B. A., Narayanan N. K., Simi B., Reddy B. S. (2003) Modulation of inducible nitric oxide synthase and related proinflammatory genes by the omega-3 fatty acid docosahexaenoic acid in human colon cancer cells. *Cancer Res.* 63:972-979.

[103] Nitenberg G. (2000) Nutritional support in sepsis: still skeptical? *Curr.Opin.Crit Care* 6:253-266.

[104] Pacht E. R., DeMichele S. J., Nelson J. L., Hart J., Wennberg A. K., Gadek J. E. (2003) Enteral nutrition with eicosapentaenoic acid, gamma-linolenic acid, and antioxidants reduces alveolar inflammatory mediators and protein influx in patients with acute respiratory distress syndrome. *Crit Care Med.* 31:491-500.

[105] Palombo J. D., DeMichele S. J., Boyce P. J., Lydon E. E., Liu J. W., Huang Y. S., Forse R. A., Mizgerd J. P., Bistrian B. R. (1999) Effect of short-term enteral feeding with eicosapentaenoic and gamma-linolenic acids on alveolar macrophage eicosanoid synthesis and bactericidal function in rats. *Crit Care Med.* 27:1908-1915.

[106] Poeze M., Ramsay G., Buurman W. A., Greve J. W., Dentener M., Takala J. (2002) Increased hepatosplanchnic inflammation precedes the development of organ dysfunction after elective high-risk surgery. *Shock* 17:451-458.

[107] Pontes-Arruda A (2005) The effects of enteral feeding with eicosapentaenoic acid, gamma linolenic acid and antioxidants in patients with sepsis. *Crit Care* 9:P363.

[108] Pscheidl E., Schywalsky M., Tschaikowsky K., Boke-Prols T. (2000) Fish oil-supplemented parenteral diets normalize splanchnic blood flow and improve killing of translocated bacteria in a low-dose endotoxin rat model. *Crit Care Med.* 28:1489-1496.

[109] Pscheidl E. M., Wan J. M., Blackburn G. L., Bistrian B. R., Istfan N. W. (1992) Influence of omega-3 fatty acids on splanchnic blood flow and lactate metabolism in an endotoxemic rat model. *Metabolism* 41:698-705.

[110] Robinson D. R., Xu L. L., Tateno S., Guo M., Colvin R. B. (1993) Suppression of autoimmune disease by dietary n-3 fatty acids. *J.Lipid Res.* 34:1435-1444.

[111] Rogers S., James K. S., Butland B. K., Etherington M. D., O'Brien J. R., Jones J. G. (1987) Effects of a fish oil supplement on serum lipids, blood pressure, bleeding time, haemostatic and rheological variables. A double blind randomised controlled trial in healthy volunteers. *Atherosclerosis* 63:137-143.

[112] Ross J. A., Moses A. G., Fearon K. C. (1999) The anti-catabolic effects of n-3 fatty acids. *Curr.Opin.Clin.Nutr.Metab Care* 2:219-226.

[113] Schauder P., Rohn U., Schafer G., Korff G., Schenk H. D. (2002) Impact of fish oil enriched total parenteral nutrition on DNA synthesis, cytokine release and receptor expression by lymphocytes in the postoperative period. *Br.J.Nutr* 87 Suppl 1:S103-S110.

[114] Senkal M., Mumme A., Eickhoff U., Geier B., Spath G., Wulfert D., Joosten U., Frei A., Kemen M. (1997) Early postoperative enteral immunonutrition: clinical outcome and cost-comparison analysis in surgical patients. *Crit Care Med.* 25:1489-1496.

[115] Sheth K.Bankey P. (2001) The liver as an immune organ. *Curr.Opin.Crit Care* 7:99-104.

[116] Shimokawa H.Vanhoutte P. M. (1988) Dietary cod-liver oil improves endothelium-dependent responses in hypercholesterolemic and atherosclerotic porcine coronary arteries. *Circulation* 78:1421-1430.

[117] Shou J., Lappin J., Minnard E. A., Daly J. M. (1994) Total parenteral nutrition, bacterial translocation, and host immune function. *Am.J.Surg.* 167:145-150.

[118] Sperling R. I., Robin J. L., Kylander K. A., Lee T. H., Lewis R. A., Austen K. F. (1987) The effects of N-3 polyunsaturated fatty acids on the generation of platelet-activating factor-acether by human monocytes. *J.Immunol.* 139:4186-4191.

[119] Swails W. S., Bell S. J., Bistrian B. R., Lewis E. J., Pfister D., Forse R. A., Kelly S., Blackburn G. L. (1993) Fish-oil-containing diet and platelet aggregation. *Nutrition* 9:211-217.

[120] Swank G. M.Deitch E. A. (1996) Role of the gut in multiple organ failure: bacterial translocation and permeability changes. *World J.Surg.* 20:411-417.

[121] Taniguchi T., Koido Y., Aiboshi J., Yamashita T., Suzaki S., Kurokawa A. (1999) Change in the ratio of interleukin-6 to interleukin-10 predicts a poor outcome in patients with systemic inflammatory response syndrome. *Crit Care Med.* 27:1262-1264.

[122] Tashiro T., Yamamori H., Takagi K., Hayashi N., Furukawa K., Nakajima N. (1998) n-3 versus n-6 polyunsaturated fatty acids in critical illness. *Nutrition* 14:551-553.

[123] Thijs L. G., Hack C. E., Strack van Schijndel R. J., Nuijens J. H., Wolbink G. J., Eerenberg-Belmer A. J., van der, V, Wagstaff J. (1990) Activation of the complement system during immunotherapy with recombinant IL-2. Relation to the development of side effects. *J.Immunol.* 144:2419-2424.

[124] Tisdale M. J. (1996) Inhibition of lipolysis and muscle protein degradation by EPA in cancer cachexia. *Nutrition* 12:S31-S33.

[125] Tsekos E., Reuter C., Stehle P., Boeden G. (2004) Perioperative administration of parenteral fish oil supplements in a routine clinical setting improves patient outcome after major abdominal surgery. *Clin.Nutr.* 23:325-330.

[126] Tsutsui S., Moriguchi S., Morita M., Kuwano H., Matsuda H., Mori M., Matsuura H., Sugimachi K. (1992) Multivariate analysis of postoperative complications after esophageal resection. *Ann.Thorac.Surg.* 53:1052-1056.

[127] Vainio H. (2001) Is COX-2 inhibition a panacea for cancer prevention? *Int.J.Cancer* 94:613-614.

[128] van den Berghe G., Wouters P., Weekers F., Verwaest C., Bruyninckx F., Schetz M., Vlasselaers D., Ferdinande P., Lauwers P., Bouillon R. (2001) Intensive insulin therapy in the critically ill patients. *N.Engl.J.Med.* 345:1359-1367.

[129] Vincent J. L., Spapen H., Bakker J., Webster N. R., Curtis L. (2000) Phase II multicenter clinical study of the platelet-activating factor receptor antagonist BB-882 in the treatment of sepsis. *Crit Care Med.* 28:638-642.

[130] Waitzberg D. L., Lotierzo P. H., Logullo A. F., Torrinhas R. S., Pereira C. C., Meier R. (2002) Parenteral lipid emulsions and phagocytic systems. *Br.J.Nutr.* 87 Suppl 1:S49-S57.

[131] Wallace F. A., Neely S. J., Miles E. A., Calder P. C. (2000) Dietary fats affect macrophage-mediated cytotoxicity towards tumor cells. *Immunol.Cell Biol.* 78:40-48.

[132] Weber P. C. (1990) Fish oil fatty acids and cardiovascular function: epidemiology and biochemical mechanisms. *Biochem.Soc.Trans.* 18:1045-1049.

[133] Weiss G., Meyer F., Matthies B., Pross M., Koenig W., Lippert H. (2002) Immunomodulation by perioperative administration of n-3 fatty acids. *Br.J.Nutr.* 87 Suppl 1:S89-S94.

[134] Whitehouse A. S., Smith H. J., Drake J. L., Tisdale M. J. (2001) Mechanism of attenuation of skeletal muscle protein catabolism in cancer cachexia by eicosapentaenoic acid. *Cancer Res.* 61:3604-3609.

[135] Whiteside T. L., Bryant J., Day R., Herberman R. B. (1990) Natural killer cytotoxicity in the diagnosis of immune dysfunction: criteria for a reproducible assay. *J.Clin.Lab Anal.* 4:102-114.

[136] Wolfe B. M., Walker B. K., Shaul D. B., Wong L., Ruebner B. H. (1988) Effect of total parenteral nutrition on hepatic histology. *Arch.Surg.* 123:1084-1090.

[137] Ziegler E. J., Fisher C. J., Jr., Sprung C. L., Straube R. C., Sadoff J. C., Foulke G. E., Wortel C. H., Fink M. P., Dellinger R. P., Teng N. N.,. (1991) Treatment of gram-negative bacteremia and septic shock with HA-1A human monoclonal antibody against endotoxin. A randomized, double-blind, placebo-controlled trial. The HA-1A Sepsis Study Group. *N.Engl.J.Med.* 324:429-436.

In: Omega 3 Fatty Acids in Clinical Nutrition
Editors: A. Heller, S. Stehr and T. Koch, pp. 77-88
ISBN 1-59454-601-0

Chapter IV

Omega-3 Fatty Acids and Diagnosis-Related Clinical Outcome

Axel R. Heller, Sebastian N. Stehr and Thea Koch

4.1. Background

Various strategies to control the excessive production of pro-inflammatory lipid mediators have been evaluated in numerous diseases. Inhibition of phospholipase A_2, the enzyme catalysing aracidonic acid release, the blockade of cyclooxygenase- and lipoxygenase enzymes as well as the development of receptor antagonists against platelet-activating factor and leukotrienes have been assessed (see chapter 2). However, effector cell reactions are not determined by the concentration of a single cytokine or acute-phase reactant, but by the interaction of an array of mediators. Accordingly, monocausal therapeutic interventions remain ineffectual if redundant inflammatory signals are transmitted and blocked pathways are bypassed. In addition, an up-regulation of corresponding receptors may enable signal transduction despite low signal density. For a beneficial modulation of immunological reactions it appears essential to use substances such as FO which effect not only one target but a broad spectrum of signals in favor of patient homeostasis.

Apart from supplying energy, omega-3 FA generate immune-modulating and organ-protective effects. A large body of experimental data confirms that omega-3 FA attenuate inflammatory reactions, ameliorate host defense, improve capillary blood flow and gut barrier function in septic states, and prevent tumor growth.

The basis for these beneficial effects is the reduced release of pro-inflammatory arachidonic acid- derivatives. Further, inhibition of the pro-inflammatory axis of toll-like receptor 4- NFκB-axis on various levels is considered to be the molecular background of these immunomodulating effects of omega-3 FA or their respective oxidation products.

In animal experiments Pscheidl and colleagues demonstrated an improved splanchnic perfusion and a higher lactate clearance in the liver after omega-3 FA [24]. In addition, they provided evidence for enhanced hepatic immune competence in terms of bactericidal capacity after FO administration during endotoxemia [23], which can be explained by a diminished overstimulation of TLR-4 and its inflammatory downstream cascade. These circumstances may be the key factor in the improvement of liver and pancreas function after FO administration in patients undergoing major abdominal surgery [7].

4.2. Interpretation of Current Data

In recent years research activities in clinical nutrition have focused on immunonutrients, such as omega-3 FA, nucleotides and arginine [10]. The results of these studies are, however, controversial [1,2]. One of the key problems in understanding the current body of data is that most studies were carried out on a mix of immuno- active substances. Therefore, conclusions regarding the contribution of single substrates to the observed beneficial sum effects cannot be drawn. In addition, it appears that the noted effects of substances are strongly related to the patient's basic disease (i.e. critically ill vs. postoperative) or the choice of specific outcome parameters. While arginine has favorable effects on the healing process of postoperative wounds, concerns have, in particular, been raised regarding cardiovascular distress by NO-mediated vasodilatation in septic shock [9,11].

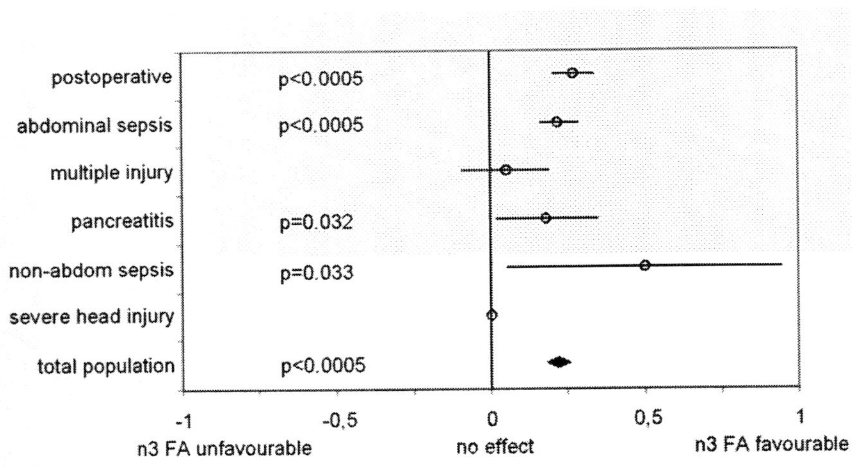

Figure 29. Effect of supplementation with omega-3 fatty acids on reduction of infections in diagnoses-subgroups as judged by the attending physician. Mean and 95% confidence intervals

Data regarding dose-dependent effects of omega-3 FA on diagnosis- and organ-failure related outcome are missing. Therefore our group addressed this problem in a prospective, open label, multicenter trial involving 661 patients receiving parenteral FO. We evaluated survival, length of ICU-stay, hospital stay, and use of antibiotics with respect to the primary diagnosis and extent of organ dysfunction. We chose a five-step approach in which we, at the very beginning, identified an outcome- relevant parameter for the dosage of omeg-3 FA. In recent publications the ratio of omega-3/ omeg-6 FA is considered a relevant dosage criterion.

Table 11. Patients' subgroup characteristics regarding the primary diagnosis
Patient mortality as predicted by the Simplified Acute Physiology Score II

primary diagnoses	n	SAPS II mortality [%]	ICU stay [d]	hospital stay [d]	fish oil dose [g/kg/d]
abdominal surgery	252	7.8±11.0	8.7±10.4	27.4±12.9	0.13±0.07
abdominal sepsis	274	21.7±16.7	13.9±17.0	30.1±20.9	0.10±0.06
non abdominal sepsis	18	24.3±17.1	19.7±12.2	34.7±16.7	0.12±0.08
multiple injury	59	46.2±26.1	22.6±19.2	38.0±29.1	0.12±0.07
severe head injury	19	52.7±17.3	13.5±8.2	20.7±13.4	0.13±0.06
Other	39	11.2±13.5	8.9±6.9	20.4±9.7	0.09±0.07
Total	661	18.9±20.0	12.5±14.8	29.1±18.7	0.11±0.07

In a multivariate analysis of multiple outcome- endpoints (mortality, length of ICU/ hospital stay, Antibiotic demand, etc.), however, the absolute weight adjusted FO dosage per day had a 2-20-fold higher predictive value on the respective outcome compared to the n3/n6 ratio. Thus we used this parameter for further analysis. The second step was the evaluation of dose-related effects on the entire study cohort, which was then in a third and a fourth step broken down to diagnosis and organ-failure-related outcome, respectively. The final step allowed definite assumptions on the diagnosis- or organ failure-related optimum dosage of FO using a polynomial curve fit.Fish oil supplementation had dose-dependent beneficial effects on the observed outcome parameters.

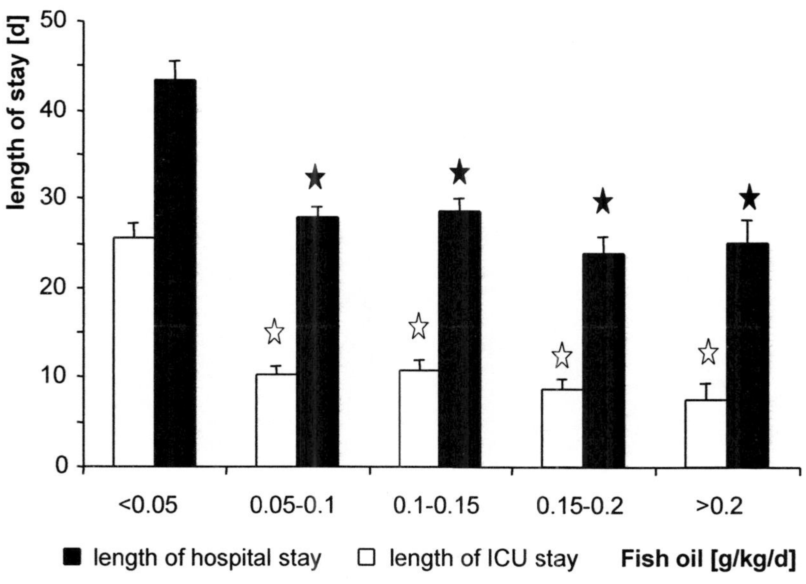

Figure 30. Dose-related length of stay (mean and SEM) black columns in hospital, white columns in ICU. Between- group comparisons are SAPS II and mortality adjusted in statistical analysis White asterisk ICU stay p<0.001 vs. dose lower than 0.05g/kg/d; black asterisk hospital stay p<0.001 vs. dose lower than 0.05g/kg/d

Compared to the subgroup receiving less than 0.05g/kg/d of omega 3 FA significantly more patients survived when 0.1-0.2 g/kg/d were administered. Furthermore, doses exceeding 0.05g/kg/d were sufficient to shorten the length of both, ICU and hospital stay (figure 30). This observation may be attributed to the lower requirement of antibiotic treatment when omega-3 FA were given in daily doses between 0.15 and 0.2 g/kg (figure 31).

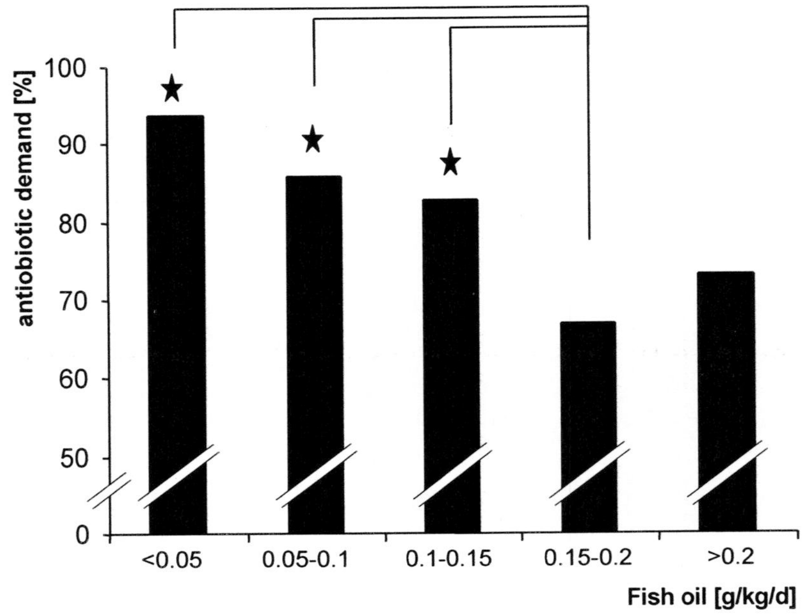

Figure 31. Antibiotic demand in percent of patients in dose-related subgroups. Asterisk $p<0.05$

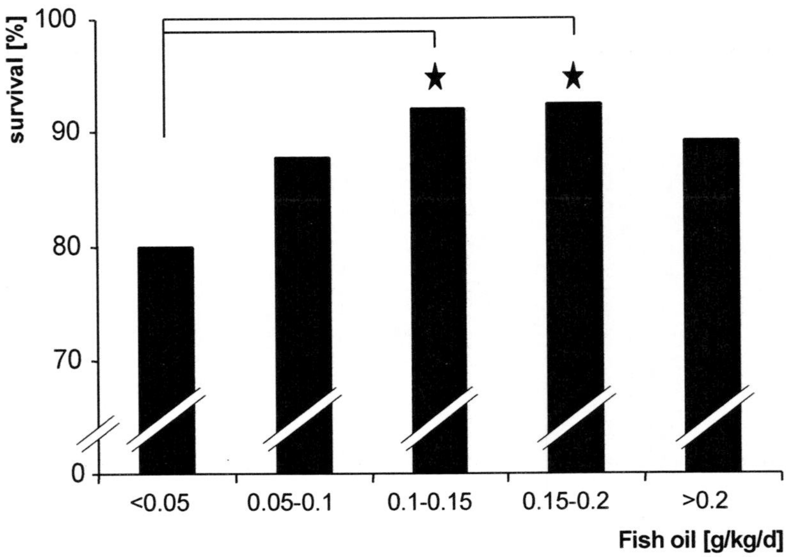

Figure 32. Survival in percent of patients in dose-related subgroups. Asterisk $p<0.01$

The improved condition of the patients receiving doses of FO between 0.1 and 0.2 g/kg/d is, likewise, impressively reflected by improved survival (figure 32). As previously discussed, these observations are in accordance with recent published results [3,27] and are in line with experimental data by Kelbel [13] and Pscheidl [23] who found improved bactericidal activity in animals treated with omega-3 FA. The latter results were confirmed by Weiss in a randomized trial involving postoperative patients [28]. After a perioperative administration of 10g/d of FO patients had less severe infections due to reduced immune suppression as evidenced by elevated HLA-DR- levels. In addition, a shorter ICU- and hospital stay was observed in the FO group.

4.3. Postoperative Patients

It has been shown that even a short-term parenteral nutrition with fish oil increased EPA and DHA in leukocyte [20] and platelet membrane phospholipids in postoperative patients [25] and during sepsis [17]. The decreased ratio of omega-6 to omega-3 FA in membrane phospholipids was associated with an altered lipid mediator and cytokine production. A parenteral nutrition based on fish oil and fed to postoperative patients for three days reduced LPS-induced IL-1 release and thromboxane B_2 generation and was associated with a clinical reduction of sepsis incidence [14]. These results among surgical patients are in close agreement with those obtained from patients with active Crohn´s disease [12] and cancer patients [26]. Further, patients having been treated with fish oil and undergoing major surgery have a less inhibited cell-mediated immunity and coagulation and other platelet functions were not negatively influenced by fish oil infusion [6,7]. The down-regulation of the overshooting inflammatory response, and, simultaneously, a smaller postoperative immune suppression after 10g/d fish oil was associated with less severe infections [28]. In addition, a shorter ICU- and hospital stay was observed [7,14,28] and an accelerated normalization of liver and pancreas enzymes after perioperative fish oil supplementation in patients at risk for sepsis was documented [7].

Further evidence of the beneficial effects of omega-3 FA was provided by 661 patients receiving omega-3 FA in different quantities with a subgroup of 252 postoperative surgical patients. As expected, depending on the dosage, the infection rate was significantly lower (figures 29&31) [15]. Patients who received at least 5% of the daily caloric intake in form of fish oil had a lower demand of antibiotics within the observation period. Postoperative patients had a shorter length of hospital stay. Likewise, there were fewer complications under fish oil supplementation, as was anticipated. Moreover, evaluation of the patient's clinical course turned out more advantageous. Further analysis of this cohort revealed distinct beneficial dose- and diagnosis-related effects of omega-3 FA on clinical outcome. Omega-3 FA dose optimization around 0.15g/kg/d reduced ICU- stay from 8.7 to 5.3 days and hospital stay from 27.4 to 25.5 days, respectively. Based on these data parenteral nutrition with omega-3 FA can also be termed as a cost effective treatment. These results clearly demonstrate the clinically relevant beneficial effects of omega-3 fatty acids on clinical outcome after major abdominal surgery.

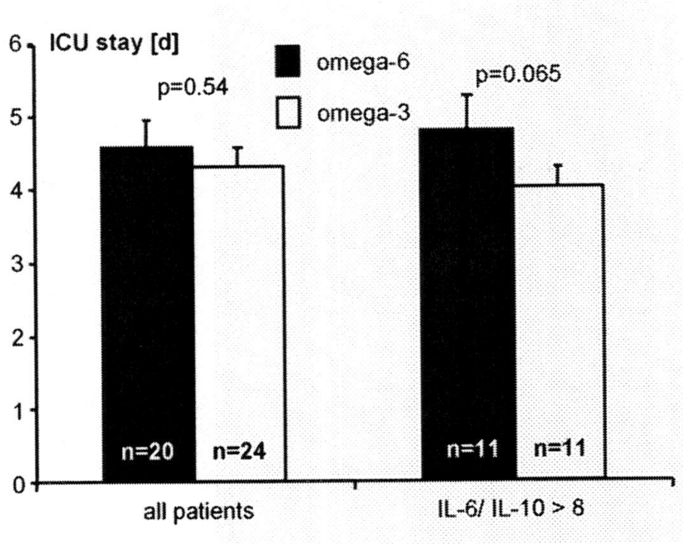

Figure 33. ICU stay comparison between fish oil and soy oil application. All patients and patients at risk for sepsis. (Reprinted with permission, International Journal of Cancer © copyright (2004) Wiley-Liss Inc., from Heller AR, et al.)

Mortality among the postoperative patients or those without organ failure did not differ regarding the quantity of omega-3 FA dose, which evidently can be explained by the (fortunately) low *a priori* mortality in postoperative patients. The lower the *a priori* mortality in a cohort, the lower are the potential significant effects of an intervention on the absolute mortality. This effect applies to postoperative patients and to those without organ failure, even when the observed subpopulations are relatively large [8].

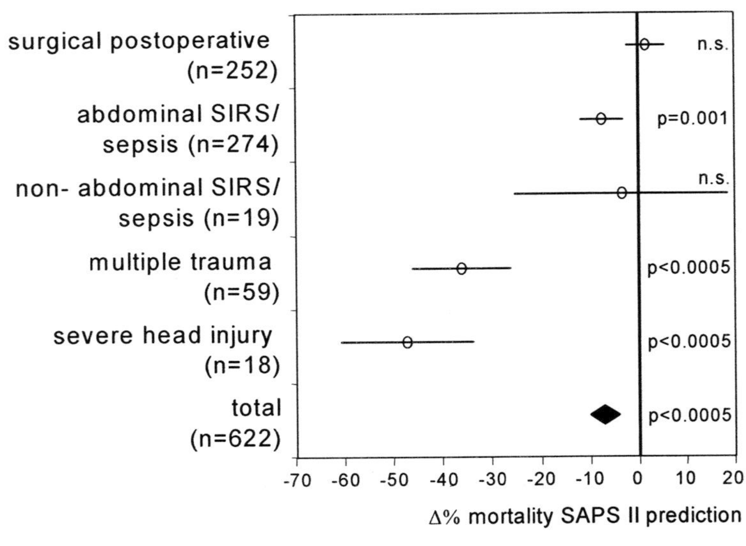

Figure 34. Diagnoses-related difference between SAPS II predicted mortality (equals 0, y-axis) and observed mortality (mean and 95% confidence intervals) Absolute mortality and FO doses can be taken from table 11. P values given for Wald test for differences: 0 equals no effect = same mortality as predicted.

4.4. Peritonitis and Abdominal Sepsis

Although data on *ex vivo*-stimulated cells from septic patients receiving FO have been reported by Mayer and Grimminger [17,18,19] virtually no research exists regarding the effect of omega 3 FA on clinical outcome in peritonitis and abdominal sepsis. Most recently, first randomized preliminary reports [3,22] demonstrate favorable effects of omega-3 FA fish oil supplementation on survival in critically ill patients. A fish oil supplementation over five days given to 54 patients with abdominal sepsis [3] reduced CRP-levels, an indicator of the inflammatory reaction. Moreover, lower re-operation rates were found and ICU- as well as hospital stay was significantly reduced in the fish oil group. Preliminary data by Pontes-Arruda indicate significantly lower ventilatory support, lower ICU-stay and improved survival in 30 patients with sepsis and septic shock [22] after enteral omega-3 FA. Moreover Tsekos retrospectively analyzed the effects of routine peri- and postoperative parenteral applications of fish oil supplements on 249 ICU patients [27]. The results again clearly indicate that the perioperative provision of parenteral fish oil (10g/day) beneficially influences patient outcome in terms of decreased hospital mortality, requirement of postoperative mechanical ventilation and hospital stay.

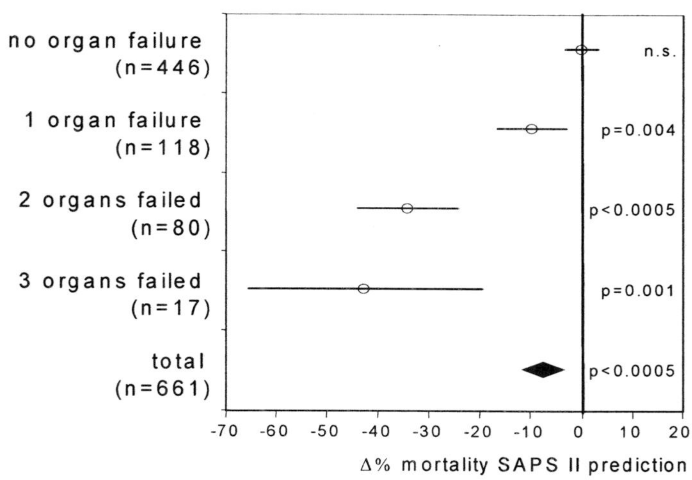

Figure 35. Organ failure-related difference between SAPS II predicted mortality (equals 0, y-axis) and observed mortality (mean and 95% confidence intervals). Absolute mortality and FO doses can be taken from table 11. P values given for Wald test for differences: 0 equals no effect = same mortality as predicted.

These results are well in line with those of the trial mentioned previously involving 661 patients including 274 patients with abdominal sepsis (figure 34) receiving parenteral fish oil who, likewise, had lower infection rates and a reduced length of hospital stay [8,15].

On closer scrutiny the predicted mortality by the SAPS II- score [16] was 21.7%. The actual mortality in this group, however, was substantially reduced by 7.4 % (CI_{95} 3.1-11.8). Optimum doses sufficient to reduce ICU- and hospital stay in diagnoses subgroups can be taken from table 12.

Table 12. Optimum doses of fish oil and respective effects on outcome in diagnoses subgroups. [a]Inverse linear correlation between length of stay and omega-3 fatty acid dose (the higher the dose, the lower length of stay). [b] Regression models not valid as indicated.

	ICU stay		hospital stay	
	Fish oil [g/kg/d]	R^2	Fish oil [g/kg/d]	R^2
total study population	0.30	0.44	0.26	0.11
abdominal sepsis	0.23	0.44	0.17	0.26
abd. surgery postoperative	linear[a]	0.27	[b]	-
No organ failure	[b]	-	linear[a]	0.13
1 organ failure	[b]	-	0.14	0.24

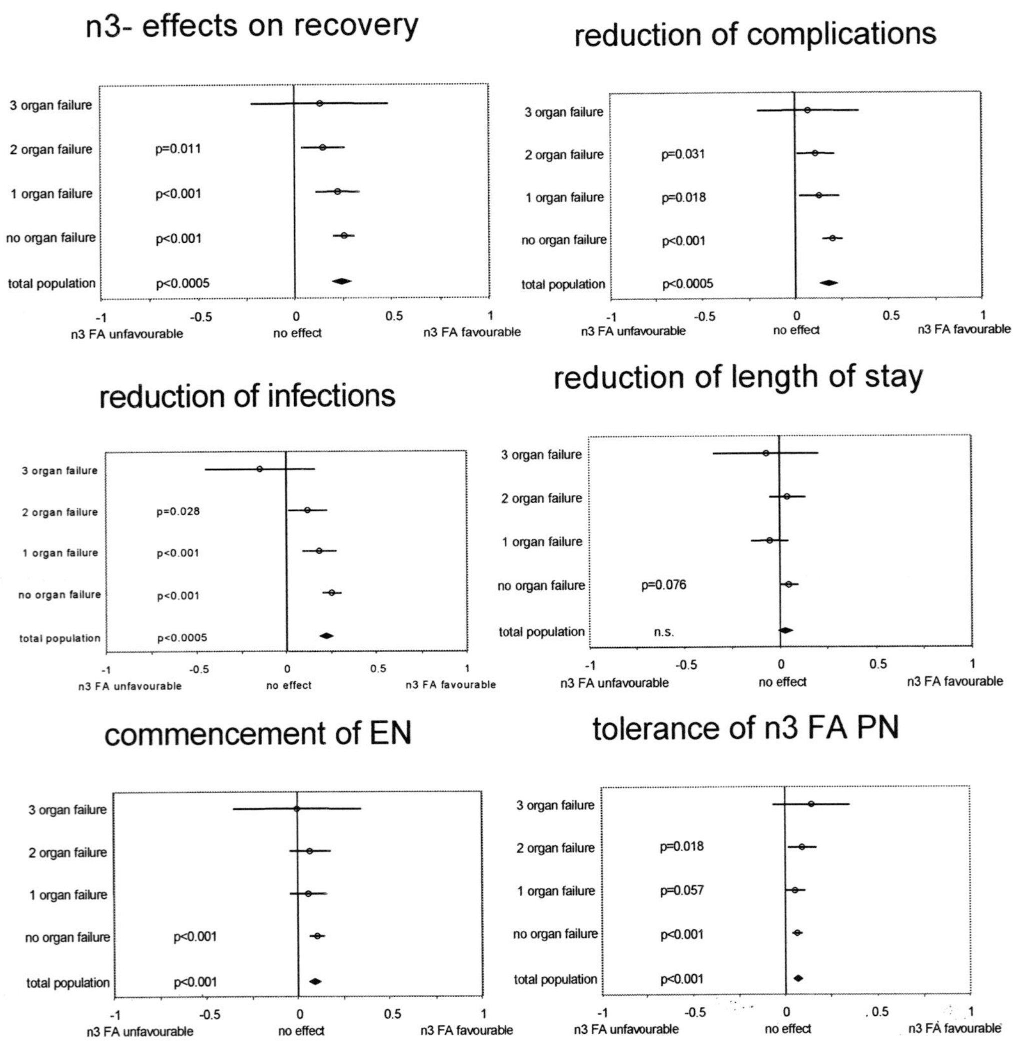

Figure 36. Effect of supplementation with omega-3 fatty acids on global recovery of the patient, reduction of complications of any cause, reduction of infections, reduction of length of stay, the commencement of enteral nutrition (EN), and tolerance of parenteral (PN) omega-3 lipid emulsion in organ failure subgroups as judged by the attending physician. Data taken from [8,15].

Besides the diagnosis-related analyses of this work [8], the scrutiny of omega-3 FA effects in different stages of organ failure seemed worthwhile. Based upon the predicted mortality by SAPS II [16] the mean administered doses of 0.10-0.11 g/kg/d fish oil were sufficient to substantially reduce mortality, length of ICU and hospital stay in patients with one to three failed organs. The fact, that mortality was not changed in patients without organ failure (figure 35) must be attributed to the circumstance that regarding postoperative patients the *a priori* mortality is too low for any single intervention to substantially lower it further.

4.5. What is the Impact of the Ratio of Omega-3/6 Fatty Acids on Outcome?

Recent literature discusses the ratio of omega 3/ omega 6 FA as a key factor affecting the immunoregulatory potential of intravenous fat emulsions in vivo [4]. In emulsions based on soybean oil the ratio of omega-3 to omega-6 FA is approximately 1 : 7. Fish oil emulsions have a ratio of omega-3 to omega-6 FA of 7.5 : 1. Omega 3 FA compete for inclusion in cell membranes and result in the production of lipid mediators of differing potency, whereby omega-6 derived inflammatory mediators are more potent than those from omega-3 FA. In postoperative patients infused with mixtures of soybean and fish oil amounting to omega-6 and omega-3 FA ratios ranging from 6.75:l to 0.08:1, the ratio of production of lower potency to higher potency leukotrienes, by neutrophils, was highest when a mixture of 2 : 1 was given [21]. It was therefore concluded that ideal lipid solutions can be designed by adjusting the ratio of omega-3, omega-6 and monounsaturated FA. This ratio of omega-3/ omega-6 FA is a simple parameter to shed light on the nutritional deficit of omega 3 FA in epidemiologic considerations. This parameter correlates fairly well with the uptake-dose and is valid when the absolute dietary intake of omega-3 FA is relatively low.

When differences of nutritional concepts dealing with distinct omega-3 contents are discussed, the primary assumption of a correlation between dose and relation does no longer apply. Rather, adherence to the ratio as a parameter is misleading, since it is the bioavailable dose of a pharmacological agent that usually determines its effect and not the proportion of its mixture with another agent.

Animal studies which postulated the impact of the omega-3/omega 6 ratio, infused extremely high dosages of FA (9g/kg/d). In this case omega-3 and omega-6 FA were immunosuppressive when applied as the main polyunsaturated FA source [5]. Cytokine release from mononuclear blood cells was reduced in these animals. Adjusting an omega-3 to omega-6 ratio of 1:2.1 diminished immunosuppressive effects [5].

In a multivariable analysis of 661 patients receiving omega-3 FA in different amounts the dosage-related factor with major impact on outcome was identified. The correlation between the ratio, of omega-3 to omega-6 FA and outcome was weak but existent [8]. As mentioned before, Morlion described the effects on leukotriene synthesis in surgical patients to be most favorable when an omega-3 to omega-6 ratio, of 1:2 was administered at a total fat load of 1 g/kg/d [21]. Our data inicated shortest length of stay when the n3/n6 ratio was 1 : 3 – 1 : 4 at an daily fish oil dosage of 0.3g/kg/d (figure 37) [8].

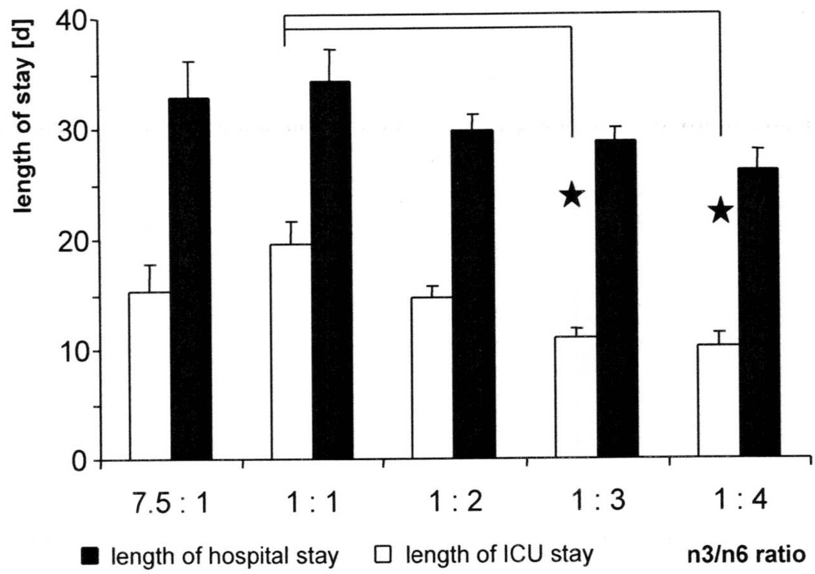

Figure 37. Omega-3/6 ratio- related length of stay (mean and SEM) black columns in hospital, white columns in ICU. Between- group comparisons are SAPS II, mortality, age, and n3 dose adjusted in Bonferroni adjusted GLM- analysis. ICU stay affected by n3/n6 ratio ($p<0.05$ vs 1:1 ratio).

4.6. References

[1] Bertolini G., Iapichino G., Radrizzani D., Facchini R., Simini B., Bruzzone P., Zanforlin G., Tognoni G. (2003) Early enteral immunonutrition in patients with severe sepsis: results of an interim analysis of a randomized multicentre clinical trial. *Intensive Care Med.* 29:834-840.

[2] Galban C., Montejo J. C., Mesejo A., Marco P., Celaya S., Sanchez-Segura J. M., Farre M., Bryg D. J. (2000) An immune-enhancing enteral diet reduces mortality rate and episodes of bacteremia in septic intensive care unit patients. *Crit Care Med.* 28:643-648.

[3] Grecu I, Mirea L, Grintescu I (2003) Parenteral fish oil supplementation in patients with abdominal sepsis. *Clin Nutr* 22:23-

[4] Grimm H., Schott J., Schwemmle K. (1998) [Development of an immuno-neutral lipid emulsion for optimal postoperative management of intensive care patients]. *Langenbecks Arch.Chir Suppl Kongressbd.* 115:599-604.

[5] Grimm H., Tibell A., Norrlind B., Blecher C., Wilker S., Schwemmle K. (1994) Immunoregulation by parenteral lipids: impact of the n-3 to n-6 fatty acid ratio. *JPEN J.Parenter.Enteral Nutr.* 18:417-421.

[6] Heller A. R., Fischer S., Rossel T., Geiger S., Siegert G., Ragaller M., Zimmermann T., Koch T. (2002) Impact of n-3 fatty acid supplemented parenteral nutrition on haemostasis patterns after major abdominal surgery. *Br.J.Nutr.* 87 Suppl 1:S95-101.

[7] Heller A. R., Rossel T., Gottschlich B., Tiebel O., Menschikowski M., Litz R. J., Zimmermann T., Koch T. (2004) Omega-3 fatty acids improve liver and pancreas function in postoperative cancer patients. *Int.J.Cancer* 111:611-616.

[8] Heller A. R., Rössler S., Litz R. J., Stehr S. N., Heller S. C., Koch T. (2006) Omega-3 fatty acids improve the diagnosis- related clinical outcome. *Crit Care Med.*38:pp

[9] Heyland D. K., Dhaliwal R., Drover J. W., Gramlich L., Dodek P. (2003) Canadian clinical practice guidelines for nutrition support in mechanically ventilated, critically ill adult patients. *JPEN J.Parenter.Enteral Nutr.* 27:355-373.

[10] Heyland D. K., Novak F., Drover J. W., Jain M., Su X., Suchner U. (2001) Should immunonutrition become routine in critically ill patients? A systematic review of the evidence. *JAMA* 286:944-953.

[11] Heyland D. K.Samis A. (2003) Does immunonutrition in patients with sepsis do more harm than good? *Intensive Care Med.* 29:669-671.

[12] Ikehata A., Hiwatashi N., Kinouchi Y., Yamazaki H., Kumagai Y., Ito K., Kayaba Y., Toyota T. (1992) Effect of intravenously infused eicosapentaenoic acid on the leukotriene generation in patients with active Crohn's disease. *Am.J.Clin Nutr* 56:938-942.

[13] Kelbel I., Koch T., Prechtl A., Heller A., Schlotzer E., Schiefer G., Neuhof H. (1999) Effects of Parenteral Application of Fish Oil versus Soy Oil Emulsions on Bacterial Clearance functions. *Infusionsther.Transfusionsmed.* 26:226-232.

[14] Kelbel I., Wagner F., Wiedeck-Suger H, Kelbel M, Weiss M, Schneider M, Grünert A, Hartung T, Georgieff M (2002) Effects of n-3 fatty acids on immune function: A double- blind, randomized trial of fish oil based infusion in postoperative patients. *Clin Nutr* 21:P39-

[15] Koch T.Heller A. (2005) Outcome-Effects of parenteral nutrition with omega-3 fatty acids - a multicenter observation in 661 patients. *Aktuel.Ernaehr.Med.* 30:15-22.

[16] Le Gall, Jr., Lemeshow S., Saulnier F. (1993) A new Simplified Acute Physiology Score (SAPS II) based on a European/North American multicenter study. *JAMA* 270:2957-2963.

[17] Mayer K., Fegbeutel C., Hattar K., Sibelius U., Kramer H. J., Heuer K. U., Temmesfeld-Wollbruck B., Gokorsch S., Grimminger F., Seeger W. (2003) Omega-3 vs. omega-6 lipid emulsions exert differential influence on neutrophils in septic shock patients: impact on plasma fatty acids and lipid mediator generation. *Intensive Care Med.* 29:1472-1481.

[18] Mayer K., Gokorsch S., Fegbeutel C., Hattar K., Rosseau S., Walmrath D., Seeger W., Grimminger F. (2003) Parenteral nutrition with fish oil modulates cytokine response in patients with sepsis. *Am.J.Respir.Crit Care Med.* 167:1321-1328.

[19] Mayer K., Grimm H., Grimminger F., Seeger W. (2002) Parenteral nutrition with n-3 lipids in sepsis. *Br.J.Nutr.* 87 Suppl 1:S69-S75.

[20] Morlion B. J., Torwesten E., Lessire H., Sturm G., Peskar B. M., Furst P., Puchstein C. (1996) The effect of parenteral fish oil on leukocyte membrane fatty acid composition and leukotriene-synthesizing capacity in patients with postoperative trauma. *Metabolism* 45:1208-1213.

[21] Morlion B. J., Torwesten E., Wrenger K., Puchstein C., Fürst P. (1997) What is the optimum n-3 to n-6 fatty acid ratio of parenteral lipid emulsions in postoperative trauma? *Clin Nutr* 16:49-

[22] Pontes-Arruda A (2005) The effects of enteral feeding with eicosapentaenoic acid, gamma linolenic acid and antioxidants in patients with sepsis. *Crit Care* 9:P363.

[23] Pscheidl E., Schywalsky M., Tschaikowsky K., Boke-Prols T. (2000) Fish oil-supplemented parenteral diets normalize splanchnic blood flow and improve killing of translocated bacteria in a low-dose endotoxin rat model. *Crit Care Med.* 28:1489-1496.

[24] Pscheidl E. M., Wan J. M., Blackburn G. L., Bistrian B. R., Istfan N. W. (1992) Influence of omega-3 fatty acids on splanchnic blood flow and lactate metabolism in an endotoxemic rat model. *Metabolism* 41:698-705.

[25] Roulet M., Frascarolo P., Pilet M., Chapuis G. (1997) Effects of intravenously infused fish oil on platelet fatty acid phospholipid composition and on platelet function in postoperative trauma. *JPEN J.Parenter.Enteral Nutr.* 21:296-301.

[26] Takagi K., Yamamori H., Furukawa K., Miyazaki M., Tashiro T. (2001) Perioperative supplementation of EPA reduces immunosuppression induced by postoperative chemoradiation therapy in patients with esophageal cancer. *Nutrition* 17:478-479.

[27] Tsekos E., Reuter C., Stehle P., Boeden G. (2004) Perioperative administration of parenteral fish oil supplements in a routine clinical setting improves patient outcome after major abdominal surgery. *Clin.Nutr.* 23:325-330.

[28] Weiss G., Meyer F., Matthies B., Pross M., Koenig W., Lippert H. (2002) Immunomodulation by perioperative administration of n-3 fatty acids. *Br.J.Nutr.* 87 Suppl 1:S89-S94.

In: Omega 3 Fatty Acids in Clinical Nutrition ISBN 1-59454-601-0
Editors: A. Heller, S. Stehr and T. Koch, pp. 89-96

Chapter V

Conclusion

Axel R. Heller, Sebastian N. Stehr and Thea Koch

5.1. Therapeutical Perspectives

In the late nineties of the past century the impact of omega-3 FA on clinical outcome was recognized and a NIH, ASPEN and ASCN consensus conference recommended further research on omega-3 FA [16]. Furthermore, the most recent recommendations of the "surviving sepsis campaign" by the *Society of Critical Care Medicine* and others [20] set the goal of devising a single concept. In the light of the "PIRO" concept therapeutic options of critical illness should be intensively investigated regarding individual PRE-EXISTING DISEASE, type of INFECTION, RESPONSE of the organism and the respective degree of ORGAN FAILURE. Our group and others have been working on the cutting edge of omega-3 FA research for more than a decade, beginning in animal models of acute illness and then further developing and introducing concepts into clinical practice. Commercially available omega-3 FA enriched solutions are available for an optimal clinical (enteral and parenteral) nutrition therapy. Data, as presented in this book, indicate definitive dose-related beneficial effects of omega-3 FA on outcome in PIRO-selected patients in various diseases. Future work will implement this concept into general practice and will diligently evaluate its effects.

5.1.1. The Gordian Knot

The key issue in the development of systemic inflammatory response syndrome (SIRS) and septic organ failure is the complex pathophysiologic sequelae which is characterized by a pro-inflammatory and simultaneous compensatory anti-inflammatory response. This, to a degree, represents a sort of chaos within the mechanisms of host response [3,2] termed MIXED ANTAGONISTIC RESPONSE SYNDROME (MARS). The net effect depends on the predominance of either anti-inflammatory or pro-inflammatory reactions and may vary time dependently. Cytokines and reactive oxygen species and their role as a trigger in systemic inflammation (SIRS) have been investigated extensively. Intensive research led to the insight, that the blockade of single mediators does not necessarily improve patient outcome. Within this context simultaneous (in part redundant) physiologic effects of different cytokines make it difficult to find one single underlying factor that can be adjusted to improve outcome. Next to cytokines and oxygen radicals, it is essentially lipid mediators which contribute to the regulation of the complex mechanisms of inflammation.

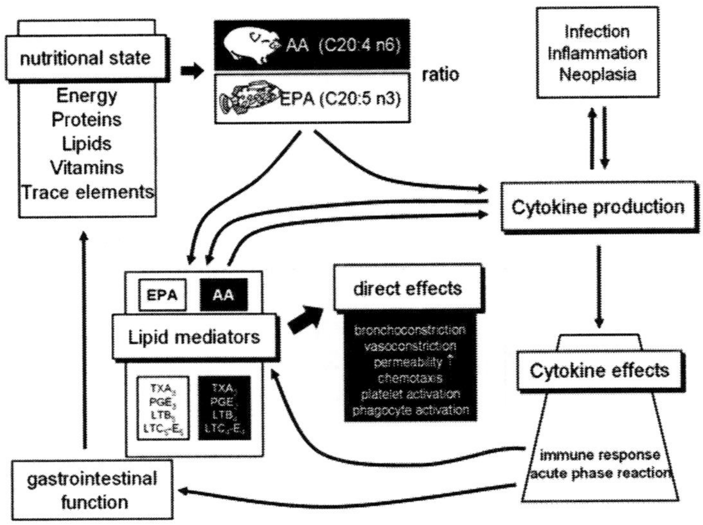

Figure 38. Effects of the omega-6 (black) / omega-3 (white) fatty acid ratio on the regulation of inflammation. The nutritional state of man is determined by the constituents of nutrition. Concerning lipids, the ratio between omega-3 and omega-6 FA determines the type and intensity of the inflammatory reaction, in terms of lipid mediators and cytokine production. While arachidonic acid (AA)- metabolites (black boxes) may induce hyperinflammation, eicosapentaenoic acid (EPA)- derived mediators are more immunoneutral Cytokine production itself as part of the acute phase response is closely coupled to lipid mediator generation via positive feed back loops e.g. by triggering the expression of COX II or iNOS. These complex interactions apply for infection and inflammation to the same degree as they do for tumor cell defense. As a result of over activated immune responses gastrointestinal function may be impaired and therefore, worsen nutritional state. (Reprinted with permission of the American Physiologic Society, from: Heller AR, et al., News Physiol Sci 2003)

Most of the studies performed with anti-inflammatory drugs did not distinguish whether the patient's condition was anergic or hyperinflammatory. Insight into the different patterns of immunological reactions during organ failure implies that the patient needs immunosuppression as well as immunoaugmentation depending on his/her individual current immunological condition. We know today that critical illness may even be beneficially modulated by augmentation of distinct defense mechanisms, while other mechanisms simultaneously have to be suppressed. The magic bullet solving this multiplicity of tasks, reducing overwhelming systemic inflammatory reaction and preventing organ failure, has still to be found. However, the effects of omega-3 fatty acids supplementation may be one key.

Table 13. Effects of dietary supplementation with omega-3 fatty acids (fish oil) in various diseases. (Modified and reprinted with permission of Adis International Ltd. Wolters Kluwer Health, Auckland, New- Zealand, from Heller AR, et al., Drugs 1998; 55(4) 487-96)

Disorder	Effect of omega-3 fatty acids
Coronary heart disease	reinfarction rate, coronary sclerosis and restenosis after PTCA decreased antiarrhathmic effects [22]
Neoplasia/ tumor growth	modulation of oncogene expression improvement of tumoricidal mechanisms reduction of cachexia [10]
Surgical patients	complications and infection rates reduced [15,17,30,31]
Peritonitis and abdominal sepsis	nosocomial infections and antibiotic demand reduced survival improved, length of hospital stay reduced [12,25]
Acute lung injury/ ARDS	decrease of capillary leakage, shorter ventilator support, earlier ICU discharge [5,24]
Bacteremia	rapid termination of experimental bacteremia and improvement of alveolar and liver macrophage activity [14]
Endotoxemia	improvement of splanchnic blood flow and bacterial killing [26,27]
Cystic fibrosis	improvement of vital capacity [21]
Rheumatoid arthritis	improvement of clinical condition [6]
Psoriasis	improvement of clinical condition [9,28]
Ulcerative colitis	improvement of clinical condition [8]
bipolar disorder	longer event-free intervals in manic-depressive disease [29]

5.1.2. Putting Pieces Together to Improve Patient Care

During the last decade pharmacological aspects of omega-3 FA have been intensively investigated and have contributed to a better understanding of the effects associated with FA administration. Besides being compact energy carriers and membrane components, lipids hold crucial functions as modulators of biochemical processes. Therefore the combination of energetic, pharmacological, and essential properties must be the object of an optimized individual nutritional concept.

Several recent studies suggest beneficial effects of omega-3 FA on recovery- and outcome-parameters in patients with major surgical interventions and in critically ill patients by lowering the extent of overwhelming self-destructing inflammatory response but at the same time improving host defense. Furthermore, increasing clinical data support the hypothesis that an optimum preoperative composition of cell membranes, before initiation of the inflammatory cascade, is more effective with respect to modulation of cytokine biology and patient recovery than mere postoperative nutrition therapy.

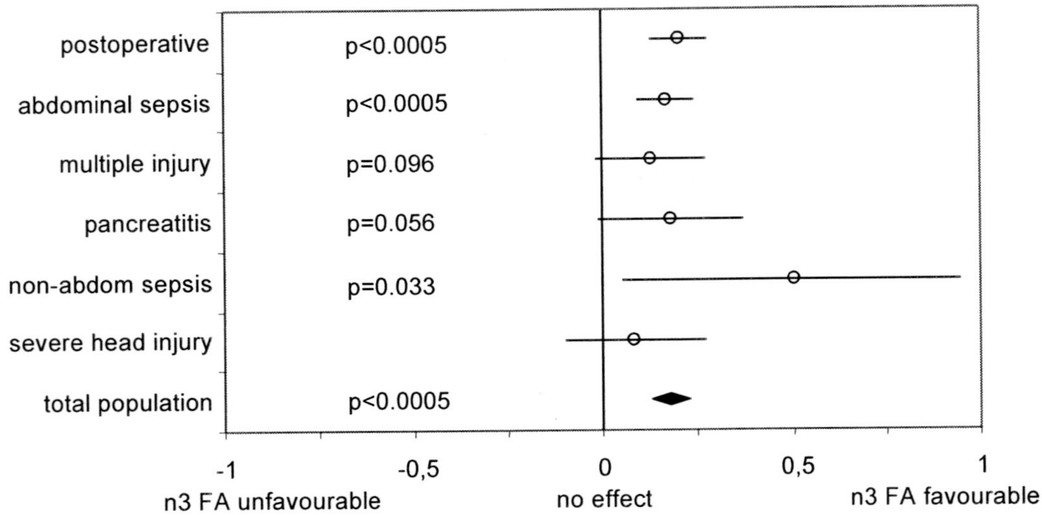

Figure 39. Effect of supplementation with omega (n)-3 fatty acids on reduction of complications of any cause in diagnoses- subgroups as judged by the attending physician. Mean and 95% confidence intervals

Accordingly, a down-regulation of the inflammatory response, and, simultaneously, a smaller postoperative immune suppression associated with less severe infections after omega-3 FA [7]. In addition, a shorter ICU- and hospital stay was observed after perioperative fish oil supplementation. Recently, Tsekos and co-workers examined a similar concept. They analyzed the effects of routine peri- and postoperative parenteral application of fish oil supplements on patient outcome [30]. The results again clearly indicate that the novel concept of perioperative provision of parenteral fish oil (10g/day) has a beneficial influence on patient outcome in terms of decreased hospital mortality, requirement of postoperative mechanical ventilation and hospital stay. Thus, in a setting of elective surgery, preoperative administration omega-3 FA appears advantageous. In the critically ill, on the other hand, early use is advisable, before complex inflammatory host actions and overshooting reactions during SIRS and sepsis commence.

Consequently, lipids should cover 30-50% of the energy demand. They can be infused after securing hemodynamic stability of the patient (about 15-30 hrs. after trauma). Isolated organ insufficiencies, are not a contraindication for lipid administration. New concepts of fat nutrition therapy should, however, aim to avoid arachidonic precursors because of a multitude of potentially adverse interactions between omega-6 FA (i.e. arachidonic acid) and immune competent cells [4]. The essential character of some fatty acids such as linolic acid (C18:3 n6) has to be kept in mind and can be taken into account by addition of medium-length FA [1]. The addition of structured lipids, including medium and long-chain FA with a faster blood clearance than physical FA-mixtures could be a further improvement [18]. Of course, fish oil should be added up to 0.1-0.2 g/kg/d [5,11,23]. Which role olive oil, a monounsaturated fatty acid, may play in the future can momentarily not be assessed. Nevertheless, an ideal fatty acid combination still needs to be defined. Future combinations administered in patients could consist of 30-40% LCTs with 40-50% MCTs (ideally as structured lipids), 15-20% fish oil and possibly 15-20% olive oil.

	postoperative patients	abdominal sepsis	non-abdom. sepsis	multiple injury	severe head injury	0-organ failure	1-organ failure	2-organ failure	3-organ failure	total
course of recovery	+	+	+	+	(+)	+	+	+	0	+
complications ↓	+	+	+	(+)	0	+	+	+	0	+
infections ↓	+	+	+	0	0	+	+	+	0	+
length of stay ↓	+	0	(+)	0	0	(+)	0	0	0	(+)
commencement of EN	+	+	0	0	0	+	0	0	0	+
tolerance	+	+	0	0	0	+	(+)	+	0	+
mortality ↓	0	+	0	+	+	0	+	+	+	+

+ beneficial ($p<0.05$) (+) probably beneficial ($p=0.05$-0.07) 0 no effect

Figure 40. Effect of supplementation with omega-3 fatty acids on the global course of recovery, reduction of complications of any cause, reduction of infections, reduction of length of stay, the ability to commence enteral nutrition (EN), and tolerance of omega-3 lipid emulsion in diagnoses- and organ failure subgroups as judged by the attending physician and reduction of mortality as predicted by SAPS II

5.2. Outlook

Supplementation with omega-3 FA improves survival and accelerates recovery. These substantial effects were shown in different diseases to a variable extent. According to the most recent recommendations [13,19,20] we found omega-3 FA to be a valuable nutritional additive to improve outcome in patients with peritonitis, trauma, abdominal SIRS and sepsis, but also to reduce infections and complication rates in postoperative patients. Regarding the poor body of literature with respect to outcome data for single substrates such as omega-3 FA, further prospective randomized double-blinded trials are required to delineate the definite value of adjunctive therapy with omega-3 FA. In particular, the investigation of dose-related effects in specific diseases is crucial to further optimize clinical nutrition.

5.3. References

[1] Adolph M. (1999) Lipid emulsions in parenteral nutrition. *Ann.Nutr.Metab* 43:1-13.

[2] Bone R. C. (1996) Sir Isaac Newton, sepsis, SIRS, and CARS. *Crit Care Med.* 24:1125-1128.

[3] Bone R. C. (1996) Toward a theory regarding the pathogenesis of the systemic inflammatory response syndrome: what we do and do not know about cytokine regulation. *Crit Care Med.* 24:163-172.

[4] Calder P. C., Yaqoob P., Thies F., Wallace F. A., Miles E. A. (2002) Fatty acids and lymphocyte functions. *Br.J.Nutr.* 87 Suppl 1:S31-S48.

[5] Gadek J. E., DeMichele S. J., Karlstad M. D., Pacht E. R., Donahoe M., Albertson T. E., Van Hoozen C., Wennberg A. K., Nelson J. L., Noursalehi M. (1999). Effect of enteral feeding with eicosapentaenoic acid, gamma-linolenic acid, and antioxidants in patients with acute respiratory distress syndrome. Enteral Nutrition in ARDS Study Group. *Crit Care Med.* 27:1409-1420.

[6] Geusens P., Wouters C., Nijs J., Jiang Y., Dequeker J. (1994) Long-term effect of omega-3 fatty acid supplementation in active rheumatoid arthritis. A 12-month, double-blind, controlled study. *Arthritis Rheum.* 37:824-829.

[7] Grecu I, Mirea L, Grintescu I (2003) Parenteral fish oil supplementation in patients with abdominal sepsis. *Clin Nutr* 22:23-

[8] Grimminger F., Fuhrer D., Papavassilis C., Schlotzer E., Mayer K., Heuer K. U., Kiss L., Walmrath D., Piberhofer S., Lubbecke F., . (1993) Influence of intravenous n-3 lipid supplementation on fatty acid profiles and lipid mediator generation in a patient with severe ulcerative colitis. *Eur.J.Clin.Invest* 23:706-715.

[9] Grimminger F., Mayser P., Papavassilis C., Thomas M., Schlotzer E., Heuer K. U., Fuhrer D., Hinsch K. D., Walmrath D., Schill W. B., . (1993) A double-blind, randomized, placebo-controlled trial of n-3 fatty acid based lipid infusion in acute, extended guttate psoriasis. Rapid improvement of clinical manifestations and changes in neutrophil leukotriene profile. *Clin.Investig.* 71:634-643.

[10] Hardman W. E. (2002) Omega-3 fatty acids to augment cancer therapy. *J.Nutr.* 132:3508S-3512S.

[11] Heller AR, Fischer S, Roessel T, Gottschlich B, Ragaller M, Tiebel O, Menschikowski M, Zimmermann T, Albrecht DM, Koch T (2001) Immunonutritional aspects of parenteral fish oil supplementation after major abdominal surgery. *Crit Care Med.* 29:A127-

[12] Heller A. R., Rössler S., Litz R. J., Stehr S. N., Heller S. C., Koch T. (2006) Omega-3 fatty acids improve the diagnosis- related clinical outcome. *Crit Care Med.* 38(4):pp

[13] Heyland D. K., Dhaliwal R., Drover J. W., Gramlich L., Dodek P. (2003) Canadian clinical practice guidelines for nutrition support in mechanically ventilated, critically ill adult patients. *JPEN J.Parenter.Enteral Nutr.* 27:355-373.

[14] Kelbel I., Koch T., Prechtl A., Heller A., Schlotzer E., Schiefer G., Neuhof H. (1999) Effects of Parenteral Application of Fish Oil versus Soy Oil Emulsions on Bacterial Clearance functions. *Infusionsther.Transfusionsmed.* 26:226-232.

[15] Kelbel I., Wagner F., Wiedeck-Suger H, Kelbel M, Weiss M, Schneider M, Grünert A, Hartung T, Georgieff M (2002) Effects of n-3 fatty acids on immune function: A double- blind, randomized trial of fish oil based infusion in postoperative patients. *Clin Nutr* 21:P39-

[16] Klein S., Kinney J., Jeejeebhoy K., Alpers D., Hellerstein M., Murray M., Twomey P. (1997) Nutrition support in clinical practice: review of published data and recommendations for future research directions. Summary of a conference sponsored by the National Institutes of Health, American Society for Parenteral and Enteral Nutrition, and American Society for Clinical Nutrition. *Am.J.Clin.Nutr.* 66:683-706.

[17] Koch T.Heller A. (2005) Outcome-Effects of parenteral nutrition with omega-3 fatty acids - a multicenter observation in 661 patients. *Aktuel.Ernaehr.Med.* 30:15-22.

[18] Kruimel J. W., Naber T. H., van der, V, Carneheim C., Katan M. B., Jansen J. B. (2001) Parenteral structured triglyceride emulsion improves nitrogen balance and is cleared faster from the blood in moderately catabolic patients. *JPEN J.Parenter.Enteral Nutr.* 25:237-244.

[19] Levy M. M., Fink M. P., Marshall J. C., Abraham E., Angus D., Cook D., Cohen J., Opal S. M., Vincent J. L., Ramsay G. (2003) 2001 SCCM/ESICM/ACCP/ATS/SIS International Sepsis Definitions Conference. *Crit Care Med.* 31:1250-1256.

[20] Levy M. M., Pronovost P. J., Dellinger R. P., Townsend S., Resar R. K., Clemmer T. P., Ramsay G. (2004) Sepsis change bundles: converting guidelines into meaningful change in behavior and clinical outcome. *Crit Care Med.* 32:S595-S597.

[21] Manner T., Guida L., Katz D. P., Askanazi J., Schlotzer E., Wiese S., Skeie B., Fürst P. (1992) Parenteral fish-oil administration in patients with cystic fibrosis. *Clin Nutr* 11:

[22] Marchioli R., Barzi F., Bomba E., Chieffo C., Di Gregorio D., Di Mascio R., Franzosi M. G., Geraci E., Levantesi G., Maggioni A. P., Mantini L., Marfisi R. M., Mastrogiuseppe G., Mininni N., Nicolosi G. L., Santini M., Schweiger C., Tavazzi L., Tognoni G., Tucci C., Valagussa F. (2002) Early protection against sudden death by n-3 polyunsaturated fatty acids after myocardial infarction: time-course analysis of the results of the Gruppo Italiano per lo Studio della Sopravvivenza nell'Infarto Miocardico (GISSI)-Prevenzione. *Circulation* 105:1897-1903.

[23] Mayer K., Grimm H., Grimminger F., Seeger W. (2002) Parenteral nutrition with n-3 lipids in sepsis. *Br.J.Nutr.* 87 Suppl 1:S69-S75.

[24] Pacht E. R., DeMichele S. J., Nelson J. L., Hart J., Wennberg A. K., Gadek J. E. (2003) Enteral nutrition with eicosapentaenoic acid, gamma-linolenic acid, and antioxidants reduces alveolar inflammatory mediators and protein influx in patients with acute respiratory distress syndrome. *Crit Care Med.* 31:491-500.

[25] Pontes-Arruda A (2005) The effects of enteral feeding with eicosapentaenoic acid, gamma linolenic acid and antioxidants in patients with sepsis. *Crit Care* 9:P363.

[26] Pscheidl E., Schywalsky M., Tschaikowsky K., Boke-Prols T. (2000) Fish oil-supplemented parenteral diets normalize splanchnic blood flow and improve killing of translocated bacteria in a low-dose endotoxin rat model. *Crit Care Med.* 28:1489-1496.

[27] Pscheidl E. M., Wan J. M., Blackburn G. L., Bistrian B. R., Istfan N. W. (1992) Influence of omega-3 fatty acids on splanchnic blood flow and lactate metabolism in an endotoxemic rat model. *Metabolism* 41:698-705.

[28] Soyland E., Funk J., Rajka G., Sandberg M., Thune P., Rustad L., Helland S., Middelfart K., Odu S., Falk E. S., . (1993) Effect of dietary supplementation with very-long-chain n-3 fatty acids in patients with psoriasis. *N.Engl.J.Med.* 328:1812-1816.

[29] Stoll A. L., Locke C. A., Marangell L. B., Severus W. E. (1999) Omega-3 fatty acids and bipolar disorder: a review. Prostaglandins *Leukot.Essent.Fatty Acids* 60:329-337.

[30] Tsekos E., Reuter C., Stehle P., Boeden G. (2004) Perioperative administration of parenteral fish oil supplements in a routine clinical setting improves patient outcome after major abdominal surgery. *Clin.Nutr.* 23:325-330.

[31] Weiss G., Meyer F., Matthies B., Pross M., Koenig W., Lippert H. (2002) Immunomodulation by perioperative administration of n-3 fatty acids. *Br.J.Nutr.* 87 Suppl 1:S89-S94.

Index

B

C

D

E

F

G

H

I

J

K

N

O

P

T

U

V

W

Z